Oncology Nurse Navigation

Transitioning into the Field

Lillie D. Shockney, RN, BS, MAS, ONN-CG

Co-Founder and Program Director, AONN+ Cranbury, NJ
University Distinguished Service Professor of Breast Cancer
Former Administrative Director, Johns Hopkins Breast Center
Former Director, Johns Hopkins Cancer Survivorship Programs
Professor of Surgery and Oncology, JHU School of Medicine
Co-Developer of Work Stride, Johns Hopkins Managing Cancer
    at Work Programs
Johns Hopkins University
Baltimore, MD

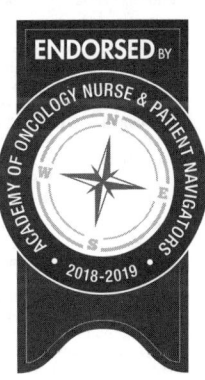

The endorsement mark certifies that the information presented in educational seminars, publications, or other resources is reliable and credible.

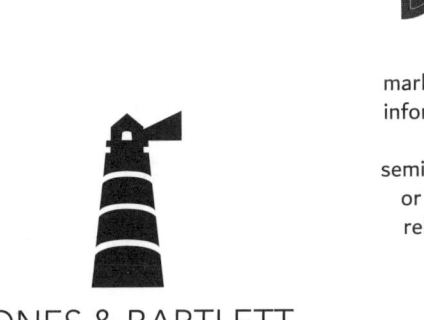

JONES & BARTLETT
LEARNING

World Headquarters
Jones & Bartlett Learning
5 Wall Street
Burlington, MA 01803
978-443-5000
info@jblearning.com
www.jblearning.com

Jones & Bartlett Learning books and products are available through most bookstores and online booksellers. To contact Jones & Bartlett Learning directly, call 800-832-0034, fax 978-443-8000, or visit our website, www.jblearning.com.

Production Credits

VP, Product Management: Amanda Martin
Director of Product Management: Matthew Kane
Product Manager: Teresa Malmberg
Product Specialist: Christina Freitas
Digital Project Specialist: Rachel Reyes
Marketing Manager: Lindsay White
Product Fulfillment Manager: Wendy Kilborn
Composition: S4Carlisle Publishing Services
Project Management: S4Carlisle Publishing Services

Cover Design: Michael O'Donnell
Text Design: Michael O'Donnell
Media Development Editor: Troy Liston
Rights Specialist: John Rusk
Cover Image (Title Page, Part Opener, Chapter Opener):
© mevoo/Shutterstock & © elena_prosvirova/Shutterstock
Printing and Binding: McNaughton & Gunn
Cover Printing: McNaughton & Gunn

Library of Congress Cataloging-in-Publication Data
Names: Shockney, Lillie, 1953- author.
Title: Oncology Nurse Navigation: Transitioning into the Field /
Lillie D. Shockney.
Description: First edition. | Burlington, MA : Jones & Bartlett Learning,
[2021] | Includes bibliographical references and index. | Summary:
"Oncology nurse navigators play an essential role in the care and lives
of oncology patients and their families. They ensure the full spectrum
of care is met with compassion and expertise for the patient, family,
and caregivers. This unique book provides new oncology nurse navigators
with the specific education and training necessary to manage all phases
of the cancer continuum, including medications, therapies, psychosocial
support, and overcoming healthcare system barriers. Endorsed by the
Academy of Oncology Nurse & Patient Navigators (AONN), Oncology Nurse
Navigator: Starting Your Professional Career covers the history of nurse
navigation, the many and varied responsibilities of oncology nurse
navigators, oncopolitics, future career expectations, and more crucial
topics to ensure a successful and fulfilling career as an oncology nurse
navigator. Written by Lillie Shockney, the President of AONN and the
modern founder of the oncology nurse navigator role, Oncology Nurse
Navigator: Starting Your Professional Career is the trusted resource for
this new and vital nursing career"-- Provided by publisher.
Identifiers: LCCN 2019036613 | ISBN 9781284198607 (paperback)
Subjects: MESH: Oncology Nursing--methods | Patient Navigation--methods |
Nurse's Role
Classification: LCC RC266 | NLM WY 156 | DDC 616.99/40231--dc23
LC record available at https://lccn.loc.gov/2019036613

6048

Printed in the United States of America
23 22 21 20 19   10 9 8 7 6 5 4 3 2 1

Contents

About the Author

Lillie D. Shockney, RN, BS, MAS, HON-ONN-CG

- University Distinguished Service Professor of Breast Cancer
- Former Administrative Director, Johns Hopkins Breast Center
- Former Director, Johns Hopkins Cancer Survivorship Programs
- Professor of Surgery, Johns Hopkins University School of Medicine
- Co-Developer of Work Stride, Johns Hopkins Managing Cancer at Work Program
- Co-Founder of the Academy of Oncology Nurse Navigators (AONN+)

Lillie D. Shockney, who has worked at Johns Hopkins since 1983, served as the administrative director of the Johns Hopkins Breast Center from 1997 to 2018 and as the director of the Johns Hopkins Cancer Survivorship programs from 2011 to 2018. A two-time breast cancer survivor, Lillie has worked tirelessly to improve the care of breast cancer patients around the world. Lillie is a published author and nationally recognized public speaker on the subject of cancer, with a focus on cancer survivorship, preservation of quality of life, metastatic breast cancer, end-of-life planning and care, and improving the cancer patient's experience. She has written 18 books and more than 350 articles on cancer care. Lillie is also editor-in-chief of the *Journal of Oncology Navigation and Survivorship*. In 2009, she co-founded the Academy of Oncology Nurse & Patient Navigators (AONN+) and has served as its program director since its inception. She is the consultant for breast cancer for national *ABC News* and *Good Morning America*, and she is also a regular contributor to *The Today Show* and *CNN*. Lillie currently serves on 34 medical advisory boards.

In 2008, the president of Johns Hopkins University and the Johns Hopkins Board of Trustees appointed Lillie to a faculty chair as a University Distinguished Service Assistant Professor of Breast Cancer. This is the first time in the history of the institution that a hospital nurse has been appointed to a distinguished service designation. She was promoted to a Distinguished Service Associate Professor of Breast Cancer in 2009. In 2016, she was promoted to full professor and is the only nurse at Johns Hopkins to have a primary faculty appointment in the School of Medicine and the only nurse to have reached the highest academic faculty ranking as a University Distinguished Service Professor of Breast Cancer.

In 2012, Lillie and a colleague created an employee benefit called Work Stride: Managing Cancer at Work. It was so successful among Johns Hopkins employees and managers that it now is offered nationally to other businesses and corporations, serving many large and midsize companies across the country. She continues her work within the Johns Hopkins Healthcare Solutions division of Johns Hopkins to enhance the program and continue to support its growth.

Lillie Shockney has received 53 national awards and 7 state awards, including Women in Business Healthcare Trailblazer Award, Johnson & Johnson's Most Amazing Nurse in America award, National Komen for the Cure's Professor of Survivorship award, and several national lifetime achievement awards. She has also been inducted into the Maryland Women Hall of Fame. Her research area of focus is preservation of quality of life for patients with metastatic breast cancer. She also does public speaking on navigation.

Currently, a documentary is being made about Shockney's life and work and is targeted for release in 2021. She tells people she never forgets where she came from—she will always be "a farmer's daughter."

Preface

I am truly excited for you! And I can't wait to meet you! You have embarked or are seriously considering embarking on a nursing career change that will open up to you the world of continuity of care; patient advocacy; psychosocial support at a truly personal level; and education for your patients and their families that will bring new meaning to why you became an oncology nurse. Even if you have been very satisfied with your current oncology nursing role and are just seeking something a little different, I promise you will not regret choosing to embark on becoming an oncology nurse navigator (ONN).

When I was writing each chapter, I found myself smiling at the computer screen in anticipation of you reading what I wrote. My hope is that you will choose to embrace the role of ONN and embark on a new chapter in your nursing career that becomes the most fulfilling you have ever experienced.

Some people, particularly those who are not intimately familiar with oncology navigation, believe it is a simple transition and doesn't require additional education, training, and dedicated experience. They are very wrong. An ONN is a nursing position like no other. It gives you the opportunity to get to know your patients and their families from the point of diagnosis through completion of their treatment or the end of their lives. I have never felt as gratified as I have in being an ONN. Even when I became the administrative director of the Johns Hopkins Breast Center in 1997, I knew I wanted to keep my finger on the pulse of the patient experience. I felt that the only way to make that possible was to continue to devote a portion of my time each day to navigating newly diagnosed breast cancer patients. I am a breast cancer survivor myself (more than 27 years now), an experience that has aided me in providing an additional level of support to my patients.

As you read this text, know that I am thinking of you and will be looking forward to personally meeting you, I hope, at a future AONN+ conference or anywhere that I am speaking to an oncology professional audience. Please make yourself known to me. I want to get my arms around you and personally congratulate you on making such a big decision to redirect your nursing knowledge and experience and to take on additional knowledge and training to become the best ONN you can be.

Remember, we see thousands of cancer patients, but an individual patient sees only one of us. Your patients will remember you forever. I know you will strive to be the best that you can be and, by doing so, you will give your patients a more positive experience as they take their journey through cancer treatment with you walking beside them.

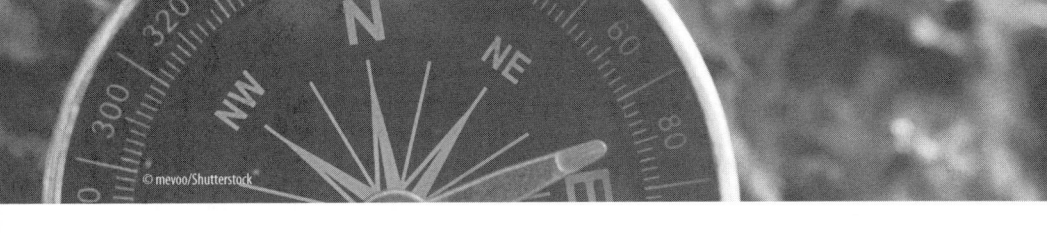

CHAPTER 1

Making the Decision to Transition from Clinical Oncology Nursing to Oncology Nurse Navigation

ongratulations on demonstrating interest in wanting to explore the opportunities that lie before you as an oncology nurse navigator (ONN)! I am so excited for you! You have already decided to make this career transition, or you want to explore this field of nursing further so you can make an informed decision for yourself and your professional future. This is not a traditionally written textbook; instead, it is a conversation between two people—you and me. I will be telling you about how to ready yourself to become an ONN, and I will be leading you on the path of success in this new role you have chosen.

An ONN is a pivotal role to fulfill as an oncology nurse while you also serve as a patient advocate. It is quite different than the role of a clinical oncology nurse (CON). I will discuss this in great detail in this text so you have a clearer understanding of what the roles and responsibilities are, how the navigation process works, and the vital importance of every cancer patient having an ONN across their continuum of care.

First, let's talk about why there is such a growing need for more ONNs across the country and the urgency that many cancer centers and cancer programs currently have to fill new or previously established oncology nurse navigation positions. An ONN is a key member of the multidisciplinary team and is often considered the hub of the wheel for the team as well as for the patients the team is caring for, diagnosing, and treating.

▶ Definition of Navigation

The Academy of Oncology Nurse & Patient Navigators (AONN+) has defined *navigation* as "the process of helping patients overcome healthcare system barriers and providing them with timely access to quality medical and psychosocial care from before cancer diagnosis through all phases of their cancer experiences."[1] The Commission on Cancer (CoC) defines *navigation* as follows: "Navigation is individualized assistance offered to patients, their families, and caregivers to help overcome barriers to care, whether through the healthcare system or the environment, and facilitate timely access to quality medical and psychosocial care from before diagnosis through all phases of the cancer experience."[2] (We will talk more about the CoC later on as well.)

▶ Goals of Navigation

The navigation goals we want to achieve on behalf of our patients fall into five categories: coordination of care, education of patients and their families, providing psychosocial support, identification and elimination of barriers by providing the necessary resources to resolve them, and always serving as an advocate for our patients. We must be forthright in focusing on providing patient-centered care and encouraging our team members to do the same. When too much focus is on the treatment, the patient can get lost, and many can forget that he or she had a life before diagnosis. Patients deserve a life during treatment and certainly a life after treatment. We need to empower our patients with educational information at their literacy level so that they can participate actively and confidently in decision making about their treatment too. Just as we hope they overcome their cancer, we must overcome the obstacles that prevent them from getting quality cancer care that is delivered in a timely manner, easily accessible, and in keeping with evidence-based treatment protocols.

Let's begin with a review of the statistics about the incidence of cancer today and what it will look like in the future. There is an increasing volume of people being diagnosed with cancer today. The American Cancer Society reported in its "Cancer Facts & Figures 2018" (available online) that 1.7 million individuals were diagnosed with cancer in 2018 in the United States. There were also 609,640 individuals who died of cancer that year.[3] According to the National Cancer Institute, as of January 2019, it was estimated that there were 16.9 million cancer survivors in the United States. This represents 5.0% of the population. The number of cancer survivors is projected to increase by 29.1%, to 21.7 million, by 2029. The number of cancer survivors is projected to grow to 26.1 million by 2040.[4]

Why the increase in those diagnosed and those surviving? Multiple reasons, when put together, explain what is happening nationally. People are living longer thanks to new methods of treating acute and chronic diseases that, in the past, would have caused death sooner. Just look at someone having a heart attack. In decades past the patient may have died; today that patient receives a stent placed to reopen blood vessel(s) in the heart so that he or she lives on for several decades. Baby-boomers are in midlife now and they are the largest population in the United States. Their numbers result in the number of people diagnosed with cancer also proportionately increasing. Midlife is the age range when most people's cancers are diagnosed. Cancer is no longer a hushed disease. We read about it in the newspaper, it is discussed in nearly every issue of popular consumer magazines, and information (good and bad) is readily available on the internet. With the explosion of social media, individuals learn through Facebook friends, online social media groups, and other means that someone they know has been diagnosed with some form of cancer. Even breast cancer, which was certainly a hushed disease a few decades ago, is now front and center with public service announcements on television promoting mammography screening and discussing the value of early detection, and documentaries about individuals who have battled and survived the disease. With more awareness of all types of cancers, more people are getting cancer screenings, which results in more people diagnosed. There are likely many people in the past who have died of a noncancerous cause, such as a stroke or heart attack, who in fact may have had cancer in their bodies somewhere but it was never diagnosed. A study done several decades ago in Sweden demonstrated that 50% of people at death have some form of a life-threatening cancer that went unrecognized. The American Cancer Society's current statistics demonstrate that one-third of the U.S. population will be diagnosed with a life-threatening cancer in their life time.[3] Staggering to think about.

With this steadily increasing volume of newly diagnosed cancer patients, there is simultaneously a growing shortage of oncology specialists. This is primarily due to medical students and residents in medical school not choosing oncology as their chosen specialty.[5] Why? The primary reason is reimbursement issues. Reimbursement for cancer care is getting more complicated, and financial coverage of the administration of cancer drugs has been reduced. Add to this the fact that more and more chemotherapy drugs are converting from IV infusions to oral administration, which patients administer themselves, and you can see that the profit margin for medical oncologists in private practice and working in the community setting has become less and less. This results in several things worthy of note: Oncology specialists have less time to spend with their patients, including with their newly diagnosed cancer patients; the ability to follow patients long term after their treatments are completed is also limited; there is a growing incidence of compassion fatigue and burnout among oncology specialists; many medical oncology private practices have actually closed their doors, choosing to retire early, or are joining a larger cancer center as a medical oncology faculty member. In such a setting, they lose their autonomy; their paycheck is usually much smaller than they were accustomed to receiving; they have many policies, procedures, and rules to follow; and the staff they work with were not selected by them. This can be a reality shock for most of these doctors making this type of transition. They are usually too young to retire, however. The final outcome can be a catch-22: More oncologists are choosing to change what they do, joining pharmaceutical companies or other physician-lead oncology organizations such as the American Society of Clinical Oncology (ASCO) or the National Comprehensive Cancer Network (NCCN), leaving what we know as the bedside. This results in even fewer oncologists staying in the clinical setting, providing care to cancer patients. Medical students and residents witness this time crunch that oncologists are forced to work in and steer away from becoming an oncologist. Seeing only patients in active treatment is emotionally draining. They miss seeing their survivors, what we sometimes call the worried well. These types of clinic visits were as much a social visit as anything. Patients thanked the doctors again for saving their lives. They reflect on the first time they met, how frightened the experience was, and so on. These patients bring joy and require little medical decision making, if any at all. Taking these patients away and replacing them with more newly diagnosed patients wear oncology specialists over time, pushing them closer and closer toward burnout.

▶ How the Shortage of Oncology Specialists Affects Your Role as an ONN

What do all the statistics mean for you, as an ONN? Your (new) role is needed more than ever. Physicians lack the time to do effective patient education and empower their patients so that they can actively and confidently participate in the decision making about their care and treatment options. Physicians are forced, due to time limitations, to focus on treatment options and not engage, as they once did, in getting to know the patient and the patient's family. The need for your position as an ONN has been growing steadily over the last decade. Where the doctors end their discussion is where you begin and, in some cases, based on the model of care you are working in, it might even mean that you do a lot of education even before the doctor enters the consultation room to see the new patient. You gather information in the process about patients and their lives that you can share with the doctor and other multidisciplinary team members. You become the touchstone for each patient and for the rest of the multidisciplinary team.

Due to insurance companies dictating where care and treatment is administered, coordination of care must be addressed as well. This is a key role and responsibility of an ONN. Patient may not be getting all of their various phases of treatment (i.e., surgery, chemotherapy, radiation, immunotherapy, hormonal therapy, etc.) in one place. There needs to be communication across the continuum of care to prevent patients from falling through the cracks. Physicians may lack the time to give a great deal of thought to what other types of referrals patients may need. Is this a young woman with breast cancer? Does she plan on starting a family or expanding her family in the future? Then a fertility preservation consultation would be needed before chemotherapy should start. It can be a narrow window of time, so it must be arranged efficiently and not as an afterthought. Is this a patient who meets the criteria for getting genetic counseling and testing? If so, the results of such a test can alter the surgical management of such a patient, switching from a lumpectomy to bilateral mastectomies. Though she works at a bank as a teller, she is actually studying to become a concert pianist, so not administering chemotherapy agents that have a high risk of causing peripheral neuropathy is imperative for her or she will forfeit her joy, her future career as a concert pianist.

As you can see, this requires knowing the patient quite well and addressing these issues before any treatment starts. We can no longer expect physicians to do this type of detailed assessment and initiate the referral process. You will be working alongside such physicians and making these recommendations, then actually arranging the referral for patients so that what needs to happen does in fact happen on behalf of each patient. We certainly want to provide patient-centered care, and your role is all about patient-centered care. Doctors also aren't in a good position to ask their patients if they have any barriers that would prevent them from getting their treatments. Again, this is a primary role of yours—identification of barriers to care and their elimination. For example, if patients don't have transportation for their treatments, they likely won't be compliant with getting those treatments. You will have access, however, to taxi vouchers and other resources to eliminate this barrier for the patients.

▶ The Common and Known Barriers to Care

Our charge as navigators is to eliminate barriers to timely quality of care throughout all phases of health care, beginning with prevention and through early detection, diagnosis, treatment, survivorship, and/or end of life. Barriers can change over time too. Transportation may be a barrier during radiation therapy, but it might not be a problem while getting chemotherapy or surgery. Barrier assessments need to be repeated, particularly when a patient transitions from one phase of treatment to the next.

Known barriers to diagnosis and treatment were identified several decades ago. They have been consistent over the years too. Although barriers to care have historically been thought of as issues that affect only underserved populations, this opinion is changing. Middle-class workers are also experiencing significant barriers. Financial barriers are steadily increasing and have an impact on most cancer patients and their families today. AONN+ has spent a great deal of time and effort in defining what the barriers to care are and how to overcome those barriers that your patients will experience. Don't feel like you have to figure all of this out on your own. Utilize this professional organization that was created with you in mind. Below are the barriers to dare as documented by AONN+ on its website.[1] The AONN+ website includes definitions and some known and reliable solutions to these common barriers. Remember that a patient can have more than one barrier and usually does. I have personally provided some examples for you as well to further define how you might utilize some of the resources available to overcome these barriers. Barriers to care can be broken down to the following categories:

- Logistical
- Financial
- Treatment
- Social
- Communication
- Emotional/physical health

Logistical barriers include transportation issues, distance from the cancer center, lack of family and/or social support, poor care coordination, and multiple appointments at different locations. Resources vary throughout the country, so it is important that the ONN have a working knowledge of local resources. ONNs can assist with troubleshooting resources and empowering the patient to think of a transportation plan to get back and forth to treatment. Transportation, by the way, is the most common barrier that patients deal with today.

Resources for transportation include the following:

- Local American Cancer Society programs
- Community transit systems
- Public transportation services
- Privates services
- Some Medicaid plans may provide transportation assistance
- Charity Air flights
- Friends, family, and community resources

Financial toxicity is a huge barrier for cancer patients and often affects a patient's decision to receive or remain on treatment. Financial toxicity refers to the way out-of-pocket expenses can drain the wallets of cancer patients, affect quality of life, and in fact become an adverse event of treatment. Patients often face high co-pays both for clinic visits and medications; face job loss as a result of their diagnosis and treatment; and are unable to meet their financial obligations, such as rent, food, and other monthly bills. In addition, low socioeconomic status affects many patients' ability to meet basic needs. If a cancer center has a financial navigator, the patient should be set up to meet this person at their first clinic visit. However, this task might also fall to you. Get creative. You might have an advocacy organization that can provide food for the patient and her family while receiving chemotherapy treatments. The patient might have money for food expenses, but maybe she doesn't have money for her co-pays or for her prescription drugs. Work with her to reallocate her food money to cover these new medical expenses and arrange for her and her family to receive food from the advocacy organization.

Financial resources include the following:

- Disease-specific organizations
- Cancer care organization
- Charity care at the point of care
- Financial advocate foundations, if available
- Pharmaceutical companies/specialty pharmacies for discount drugs
- American Cancer Society
- Chronic disease funding organizations
- Patient Advocate Foundation
- Local charitable organizations

The navigator can assist patients in overcoming treatment barriers by connecting patients with disease-specific advocacy organizations. Providing patient education and support is a large part of the navigator's role. Education regarding treatment and side effects can help patients better understand their treatment and be more compliant in care. It is important to ascertain what the patient's goals of care are and how a navigator can advocate for the patient and support those goals. This is especially important because a patient's goals may not be congruent with those of the healthcare team. Compliance issues may arise when these goals are not aligned.

Treatment-related toxicities are often a reason that patients do not adhere to the prescribed plan of care. Patients may not wish to embark on treatment or decide to stop getting treatment due to the side effects that affect their quality of life. Navigators play a key role by addressing the patient's concerns and making sure that the team is aware of the patient's side effects. Ensuring that patients are connected with the proper resources during treatment, such as a pharmacist, nutritionist, and supportive care team, can help the patient make it through treatment.

Treatment barriers may include the following:

- Lack of adherence to prescribed regimen, especially when the patient is taking oral oncolytics
- Treatment side effects
- Lifestyle/habits
- Complacency
- Lack of understanding of treatment plan
- Patients lost to follow-up care

Emotional and social barriers can manifest in many ways. Social and/or emotional barriers that impede care may include the following: age, comorbidities/sensory changes, environmental factors (smoking/alcohol use), lack of family and/or social support, poor family dynamics, mental health issues, and living conditions.

As navigators, it is important to realize that we cannot change the family dynamics, but we can try to connect patients with resources to live a healthier lifestyle, such as smoking cessation programs, counseling, and community resources for drug and alcohol abuse, and to assist them with finding a primary care provider to follow them in survivorship care. Other ancillary services, such as nutrition, physical therapy, mental health counseling, and occupational therapy, and integrative therapies, such as acupuncture, reiki, and massage, may help in obtaining a healthy lifestyle as well as managing the side effects of treatment. Calendars and written material at the appropriate literacy level and in the patient's language are useful tools to help patients.

More and more cancer drugs are oral medications that patients are self-administering, so the need for educating patients about the importance of staying on their medications as prescribed becomes a bigger and potentially harder issue. When drugs were all administered IV, the treatment may have been inconvenient for the patient, but the treatment team could be assured that patients got the treatment they were supposed to, when they were supposed to, in the correct amount, and so on. Now clinicians have lost that control. Adherence can be a really significant barrier. This can mean more phone calls to patients to discuss with them staying on track and taking their medications as prescribed.

It is important to remember the caregiver(s) too. Caregiving is hard, and many caregivers get overwhelmed. One day they were going about their life as usual, and the next they became a caregiver to a loved one while still having to continue working, taking care of children, handling the usual household chores, getting food on the table, and at some point grabbing a few hours of sleep themselves. Caregivers need additional support as well. Resources for caregivers include counseling, support groups, respite care, and connecting them with the cancer center social worker. Rarely does someone ask a family caregiver how *they* are doing. You should, but do it in private because they will likely tell you they are fine if you ask in front of the patient. Caregivers are also known for abandoning their own health and well-being while serving as a caregiver. Weight gain from not exercising and stress eating, not getting their cancer screenings that are due, and feeling guilty if they try to steal away a little time for themselves add up to unhealthy habits and a drain on health. If they are caregiving for an infinite length of time due to their loved one having advanced cancer, then caregiving is even harder because there is no light at the end of the tunnel that is welcoming. Push caregivers to do what is right for their physical and mental health, however, or there may be two patients to be taking care of before long.

Spiritual distress is a disruption of a person's belief or value system that can occur at any time in the disease course. It often surfaces at a time of stress, and it is important for the navigator to identify and understand cultural norms related to the patient's health and illness. Healthcare providers need to ensure that their beliefs and values do not interfere with care. There can even be times when, for example, in the case of a child, legal steps are taken by the hospital if parents are denying the child effective treatment due to their beliefs. Resources for spiritual distress include the following: the pastoral care department, local clergy, and the patient's clergy and support system.

Communication barriers come in many forms, such as speaking a different language, sensory changes such as visual or hearing loss, cognitive loss, and literacy issues. There is often confusion surrounding tests, medication administration, appointments, and the treatment plan. ONNs can assist in eliminating communication barriers by using translation services and providing educational materials in the patient's language that is culturally sensitive and at the appropriate literacy level. Communication must be assessed at each patient interaction to evaluate the patent's understanding of the disease and treatment, as well as to ensure that the team knows the patient's goals of care.

As nurses, we were taught to ask patients to repeat back to us their understanding of the discussion that was just held. Physicians are not taught this, however; so a physician may simply ask the patient, "You understood what I just said, right?" and the patient nods affirmatively. Sometimes, however, when you ask patients to restate in their own words what was just discussed, it becomes clear that they have no idea what the conversation was about and felt too embarrassed to ask the doctor to explain it again. Some terms may not be medical terms for patients, but in the context of a medical discussion they are and are subject to misinterpretation.

Here is an example. The doctor says to the patient regarding the fifth line of therapy for advanced cancer, "I am hopeful that your tumor will respond to this next treatment." The doctor hopes that the tumor will shrink some, but it certainly won't go away totally and the patient be suddenly cured. The patient, however, thinks that the word *respond* in this context means "cured," so she or he signs on to get the therapy, with all of its horrific side effects and financial debt associated with it, only to be disappointed in the end and perhaps even angry and feeling betrayed. The patient says, "But you told me this drug would cure me!" and the doctor responds, "I never said that." The outcome is one of distrust now, at a juncture in the treatment decision-making process that is quite profound because the next discussion usually is going to be about enrolling in hospice care when the patient was planning on a miracle drug to cure them.

So you see how barriers can have a negative impact on cancer care. The leading cause of patients not getting their treatment as prescribed is due to lack of transportation currently and it has been for years. However, financial barriers are quickly equaling and soon will surpass this barrier. Patients have large co-pays and deductibles that they are usually not aware of. When choosing their health insurance each year through their work benefits process, employees rarely read the fine print about deductibles and co-pay amounts. No one plans to have anything serious happen with their health. They might only look at what is the least amount of money that needs to come out of their weekly paycheck so that they have more cash on hand to pay their household expenses. Cancer care is more expensive than ever, however, and will likely continue to be for some time. This type of barrier, referenced above, has been nicknamed "financial toxicity" considering the financial barrier and burden to be like a side effect of a patient getting treatment.

Your clinical oncology nursing experience is helpful but won't be enough to launch into serving as an ONN.

Ideally, an ONN has at least 3 years of clinical oncology nursing experience in an inpatient and outpatient setting. The differences in the knowledge and skill set of an ONN versus a CON are noteworthy. As a CON, you took care of a patient for a snapshot of time. You may have worked in the infusion center seeing a patient only during the chemotherapy phase of treatment, and only once every two to three weeks. You were focused on safety and on appropriate administration of the right drugs, in the right dosage and at the right speed, and watching for adverse reactions and other side effects. There isn't time to sit with patients and get to know them well. Patients spend 2 hours in the infusion chair and then are gone. Education about the chemotherapy drugs may have been actually conducted by an ONN and only reinforced by the infusion nurse. If you worked in the inpatient setting, you were either taking care of patients who had had cancer surgery and were hospitalized for 2 to 5 days or were caring for patients who developed serious complications or progression of their disease, and they may die while hospitalized or be transferred to a hospice care. You only got to know them for a few days and never knew them prior to that.

A CON sees the patient for a specific phase of the patient's treatment and then may not ever see them again. An ONN, however, sees patients from the point of diagnosis (or in some cases pre-diagnosis) and continues to see patients and support them and their family members across the entire continuum of care. It is a joy to have this level of involvement and continuous interaction with your patients. You truly get to know them well, and they quickly begin to see your significant role in their lives and to utilize you as their "go to" member of their multidisciplinary team.

The charts in **FIGURES 1-1** and **1-2** compare what may be your current touchpoints as a CON compared to your new role as an ONN. Note that there is likely a different CON involved with patients' clinical care for each phase or diagnosis and treatment they experience. ONNs are more likely to be involved from prediagnosis, involved at the community outreach level with consumers, who then come in for screening, might be diagnosed, and have their treatments. Even within the treatment phases of care, patients have a different CON, and likely several of them, for *each* phase of treatment, whereas the ONN is with the patient across the continuum of care.

Being a CON is very fulfilling, but today's models of care restrict the CON's ability to really get to know patients well. For an ONN who is involved throughout patients' cancer experiences, it is a unique and often intimate relationship because ONNs enter and remain in the lives of their patients during the most critical time of the patients' lives. Patients can choose to develop a close relationship and trust their ONNs because the ONNs help them navigate from one phase of care to the next, doing their best to make the path that lies ahead efficiently orchestrated and well planned, and to involve the patient in each decision to be made.

How can you gain the training as well as improve your knowledge base to jump-start your new career into becoming a successful and effective ONN? Rely on AONN+ as a primary source for training and for networking with other ONNs who are also new or who have been in the navigation field for several years. Visit www.aonnonline.org and become a member. Save yourself a lot of time and energy in trying to figure out what the next steps are in sharpening your navigation skills. Two conferences are held each year: one is a midyear conference and the other is the national annual conference. Well over 1,000 navigation professionals attend the national conferences and, as of 2019, there are more than 8,300 members. You will be among many who are striving to continue their education, training, and even get certified as an ONN through AONN+. This organization, established in 2009, is the only national organization dedicated to navigation professionals.

I am proud to say that I am a co-founder of AONN+. It is a joy to see new navigators attending their first conference, soaking up every bit of information they

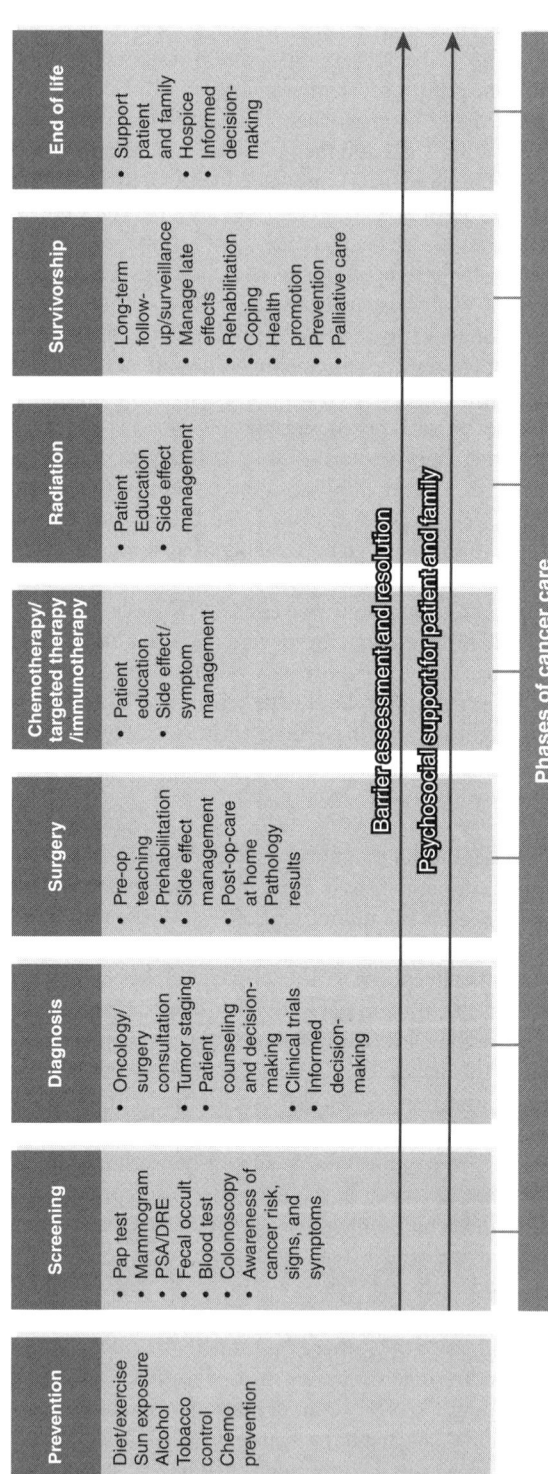

FIGURE 1-1 Oncology navigation: continuum of care.

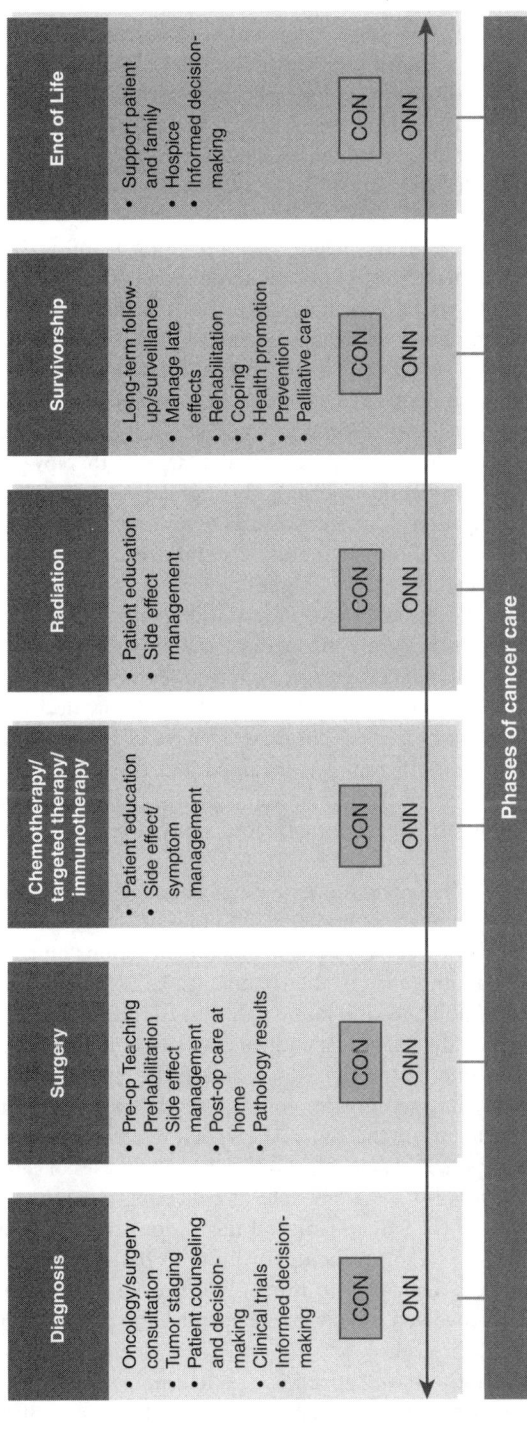

FIGURE 1-2 ONN versus CON.

can, then going home to apply it within their navigation practice. I will tell you more in Chapter 6 about AONN+ and other resources that will be valuable for you as you enter the field of oncology nurse navigation and become expert as an ONN. If your career aspirations are to advance into leadership roles, AONN+ can help mentor you with your career aspirations too. You will find specific information about this professional organization in later chapters. First, I want to provide you guidance on how to embark on what I believe will be your most fulfilling nursing career of all.

This book is intended to jump-start your knowledge and training too. A book called *Team-Based Oncology Care: The Pivotal Role of Oncology Navigation*[6] was published in 2018, and it provides you a wealth of information for you and your manager. It includes information about how to develop and implement an oncology navigation program within your institution. I was fortunate to be the editor of this textbook and a contributor of several chapters as well.

If you have worked as a CON in the past and have expertise within a specific phase of cancer treatment, such as having been an infusion nurse for several years, you will want to take some time to study about the other treatments that patients receive today, including surgery, biologic targeted therapy, immunotherapy, hormonal therapy, radiation, and long-term oral treatments. If you want to be a general ONN navigating all cancer patients who come to your cancer facility, then the void in your education may be quite significant. Take the time to study each type of cancer treated (in order of highest volume to lowest) where you are or will be working so you have some basic understanding of how each type of cancer is diagnosed; what screenings are available for early detection; how to interpret a pathology report, with all of its prognostic factors and other findings identified by the pathologist; what surgical options are available; and how decisions are made about which treatments a cancer patient may receive and why; how decisions are made about whether chemotherapy is warranted and the treatment plan that is created to give these drugs; whether radiation is part of the treatment for this type of cancer as well; and how the need for a treatment is determined as well as how it is administered.

Remember too that more and more new cancer drugs are administered today by patients or family members at home, as an oral oncolytic, which means that patients and their family caregivers need detailed instructions on administration and the importance of adherence to the treatment plan as prescribed. Although it is great that patients don't need to come to an infusion center and spend a day there, the oncology providers have lost control over ensuring that the medications are given at the right time, in the right dose, and in the right sequence, and that side effects effectively managed. Again, you can see that your educational role is paramount in helping to ensure that patients get their treatment as prescribed. You will need to know the potential side effects of each in all phases of cancer patients' treatment because you will have a key role in educating patients as they weigh the risks and benefits of each treatment and the various treatment options. It is important for patients to be given the opportunity to participate in the decision making about their care. They can do this only if they are educated about each treatment and what is involved. Involvement includes the patient's time commitment too.

What we don't want to have happen is a patient to choose to have a mastectomy for a small stage 1 breast cancer tumor that could have been effectively managed with a lumpectomy and radiation. A patient may not have transportation for radiation every day, or maybe she fears she will miss too much time from work over a 6-week treatment cycle, or maybe she assume that breast radiation will make her sick the way that prostate radiation made her dad ill, with terrible gastrointestinal-side effects that linger even today. You can see why your role is important here. You would have identified the transportation issue already and had a solution for it. You would have educated the patient about what side effects to expect from breast radiation and how different and less severe they are than what the patient's father experienced. You also could arrange to have the patient scheduled for her radiation therapy at 7:30 a.m., before she goes to work, so she doesn't miss any time from work while receiving this phase of her treatment.

If you will be specializing in a specific type of cancer, such as breast cancer, then you will be studying all phases of diagnosis and treatment for this one category of disease, and staying up-to-date about new information as it is released. You can study publications that feature evidence-based research, attend your institutions weekly breast cancer tumor board meetings, learn what clinical trials are available at any given time to this patient population, and learn what specific community resources may be available specifically for breast cancer patients.

There are also webinars provided by AONN+ and other organizations. Your cancer facility is likely already a member of the Association of Community Cancer Centers (ACCC). AONN+ has partnered with a variety of different organizations that also provide valuable educational content. We are always developing new tools and resources for our membership too. This is a very robust learning environment, so it is important that information about newly approved drugs or drug combinations from the Food and Drug Administration (FDA), new surgical methods of treatment, new radiation therapy methods, as well as new drug classifications (such as immunotherapy or CDK4/6 inhibitors) be sent to you electronically or provided in the form of seminars or conference content so that you remain at the forefront of clinical knowledge.

▶ Summary

This opening chapter has provided you with information about the genuine need for more ONNs in the oncology field. You are embarking on this new phase of your nursing career at a perfect time. The need is great, and you want to fulfill this type of significant role for your cancer patients.

The chapter included information about cancer statistics so you know the current volume and future projected volume of individuals diagnosed with cancer. I also talked about the shortage of oncology specialists, why there is such a shortage, and how we can provide to cancer patients what they need in the absence of oncologists being able to spend time with their new patients as they once could.

I discussed the definition of navigation, the goals of navigation, and how the role of an ONN is different than what was likely your prior or current role as a CON. The difference is significant. Your CON experience is vital as the baseline knowledge you need, and it will be combined with specific knowledge about nurse navigation to enable you to be the best ONN you can be! I hope too that the charts I created were helpful in comparing the CON role to the ONN role.

This chapter also contained a lot of information about barriers to care that can and likely will impede patients' ability to get screened, diagnosed, and/or treated for their cancer. Without someone to intercede, you can see why patients may not receive the care and treatment they need to overcome this disease. Much of this information that I provided comes from the AONN+ website, which I encourage you to visit.

Now let's move onto the next chapter, which is about how navigation got started in the first place.

References

1. Academy of Oncology Nurse & Patient Navigators. www.aonnonline.org. Accessed May 8, 2019.
2. Commission on Cancer. https://www.facs.org/quality-programs/cancer. Accessed May 8, 2019.
3. American Cancer Society's "Cancer Facts & Figures 2018." https://www.cancer.org/content/dam/cancer-org/research/cancer-facts-and-statistics/annual-cancer-facts-and-figures/2018/cancer-facts-and-figures-2018.pdf. Accessed May 8, 2019.
4. National Cancer Institute. https://cancercontrol.cancer.gov/ocs/statistics/statistics.html. Accessed May 8, 2019.
5. IOM Report. *From Cancer Patient to Cancer Survivor: Lost in Transition.* 2005. http://www.nationalacademies.org/hmd/Reports/2005/From-Cancer-Patient-to-Cancer-Survivor-Lost-in-Transition.aspx. Accessed May 8, 2019.
6. Shockney L. *Team-Based Oncology Care: The Pivotal Role of Oncology Navigation.* Springer Publications, 2018.

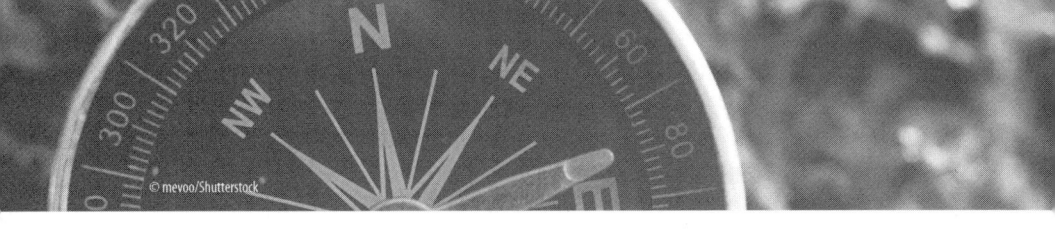
© mevoo/Shutterstock

CHAPTER 2

Starting with the Basics: The History of Navigation

This chapter starts with defining and describing the functions, roles, and expectations of an oncology nurse navigator (ONN), then it provides information about the history of this role. It is always good to know the background and history of both patient navigation and nurse navigation so that you can then understand potentially where you are headed in your professional career, as well as what it may mean for your patients in the future.

▶ Functions, Roles, and Expectations: What Are the Functions of an ONN?[1]

An ONN fulfills a critical role for many patients who have just been diagnosed with some form of a life-threatening cancer. It is not unusual for a patient to say in retrospect that she felt like her navigator was her "lifeline," her "go-to person," "her support," or "the one with the answers and solutions." If you want to become a nurse navigator or have just been requested to fulfill this role within your cancer center, you will benefit from knowing how navigation got started. It's been said that you won't know where you are going if you don't know where you have been. Your role is not just important—it is vital for the patients you will be helping in the future.

▶ What Are the Roles of an ONN?[1]

First, it's best to define a bit more what is meant by the term *navigation*. This term is loosely used today and can mean different things. It is not unusual for the leadership in your cancer facility to have requested that patients "be navigated," but they themselves are not exactly clear what they are asking you to do. What is usually meant by "navigating a patient" is that someone helps the patient move smoothly through the healthcare system, receiving the standard of care efficiently and effectively. The following is a list of roles that patients have said an ONN fulfilled for them:

- Helping me along a pathway to wellness following a diagnosis of cancer
- Scheduling tests and appointments for me
- Educating me about my treatment options and helping me figure out what happens next
- Psychological support during my treatment
- Helping me get through the maze of cancer care from surgery, chemo, and radiation to survivorship
- Making sure I don't drop through the cracks along my treatment path
- Helping me with barriers that disrupt my treatment
- Finding financial resources to help me get my treatment paid because I lost my health insurance when I got laid off
- Helping me get a cancer screening test because I had been afraid to get one before
- Helping me get in to see a doctor when I discovered I had a hard lump in my body
- Helping me find resources in my community that could assist me with child care and transportation so that I could keep my chemotherapy appointments and not miss any of them
- Matching me with a cancer survivor volunteer to talk with
- Helping me (a husband) link with hospice and other agencies to help my wife and me, actually my whole family, prepare for losing Mary

All of these statements made by patients are accurate regarding how individual patients might define their experience with navigation. It is important that you have a clear understanding of how the cancer center where you are working, most particularly the leadership of the center, defines navigation and measures your performance before you even begin your orientation for this role.

▶ What Are the Patient's Expectations of a Navigator?[1]

Whether your patient heard an ad on the radio, read about patient navigation in literature she received from someone, or simply is applying her own knowledge of what she thinks of when she hears the word *navigation*, she probably has a preconceived idea, to some degree, about what she expects you to do for and with her. Listed below are some common statements from patients describing their expectations from an ONN:

- Guide me through a complex maze of appointments, procedures, tests, decision-making steps, and actual treatment of my breast cancer.
- Reduce my anxiety about treatment by empowering me with information and reducing obstacles of concern.
- Help me overcome any communication gaps that exist between the care providers and me as well as with my family.
- Make the cancer treatment experience manageable, and help me continue to live my life during treatment as well as after treatment.

- Remove barriers impeding my care and treatment.
- Be honest with me and serve as my patient advocate.
- Represent me when there are discussions and decisions being made about my treatment options and I am not physically present to speak for myself.

▶ What Are the Cancer Center Leadership's Expectations of You as Their ONN?[1]

It is important to know what your patient may be expecting of you, but it is also important to know what your boss expects. More details will be provided about this in Chapter 5 as we look at ways to measure your success. Some common themes of leadership's expectations are listed below:

- Improve efficiency in delivery of care and treatment.
- Increase patient satisfaction.
- Reduce physician time in the clinic and on phone calls from patients.
- Ensure continuity of care and coordination of that care.
- Serve as quality control.
- Identify and eliminate barriers to care—systemically from an operations management perspective as well as individually for patients.
- Track data for quality measurement.
- Improve clinical quality and service excellence.

Do you see the importance of your role now? Does it sound like it is too hard to accomplish? It is not intended to be done alone in a vacuum. Remember that you are one member of the multidisciplinary cancer center team. Collaboration is key. There are always bumps at first while you are still learning the best way to carry out your work efficiently. The next section discusses the history of patient navigation. You might be surprised about the differences between how patient lay navigation came into being compared to how nurse navigation evolved.

▶ The History of Nurse Navigation[1]

Is an ONN a new role for clinical oncology nursing professionals? Not exactly. Let's look at the history. In the late 1970s and early 1980s, the government decided to implement major changes in how hospitals would be paid for providing inpatient care. Healthcare expenses had been recognized as being out of control even then. A patient went to the hospital the day before her operation, spent the night, and stayed in for many days afterward until she felt well enough to go home. For a woman having a mastectomy, for example, the average length of stay was 7 days. This healthcare finance system was called prospective payment, and codes were assigned to each diagnosis and procedure. In turn, specific amounts of reimbursement were provided based on the diagnosis (including comorbidities) that a patient had and the procedures she underwent. This amount of money and defined number of days allocated for the hospital stay were tied to a specific diagnosis-related group (DRG). When a patient exceeded the length of stay or maxed out the dollar limit dictated by her DRG, the hospital finance department knew it would not be receiving any additional money for the care they were providing this patient. There were some exceptions, such as specific complications or comorbid conditions that a patient might have that could bump her up to a higher-paying DRG, but the system was imperfect. If the patient was discharged prior to her designated number of days or before the threshold of the maximum payment to the hospital was reached, however, the hospital would make extra profit.

As a way to monitor this process, utilization review (UR) was conducted. UR is a process for monitoring the use and delivery of services, especially services used by a managed care provider to control healthcare costs. UR nurses were employed by insurance companies to review medical records retrospectively and determine if there had been inappropriate utilization of hospital or professional resources. Days of hospitalization that occurred on weekends when radiology services weren't available or an extra night in the hospital because the patient didn't have someone to drive her home were closely scrutinized. Doctors and the hospital received denial letters from UR departments at managed care organizations. Organizations overseeing Medicare and Medicaid (called peer review organizations [PROs]) informed doctors and hospitals that certain days of care or tests that were performed on the patient during her hospitalization would not be covered. Such decisions were often hard to reverse. Sometimes patients were discharged prematurely from hospitals because the patients had reached their DRG limit.

In an attempt to anticipate which patient's records might result in the issuance of a denial letter, hospitals employed UR nurses as well to perform the same chart review task. These individuals would inform the finance department of potential risk of financial loss based on their medical record review. In some cases, the hospital UR department also sent letters to the doctors informing them of the same and requesting that they explain why care was delivered in a less than optimal manner. The reality of the situation was that the patient had gone home and the doctor was now busy taking care of new patients. His interest in explaining why the radiology department wasn't open on weekends or why the patient requested to stay an extra day was the least of his current worries. What was more concerning were the situations in which patients were prematurely discharged and thus were provided poor care.

In the late 1980s, changes were made to this way of monitoring care, and utilization management (UM) was introduced. UM is the evaluation of the appropriateness, medical need, and efficiency of healthcare services, procedures, and facilities according to established criteria or guidelines and under the provisions of an applicable health benefits plan. Although the overarching goal, according to the U.S. Federal government and managed care organizations, was to help ensure patients were provided cost effective, efficient, high-quality, medically necessary care, the managed care organizations as well as government PROs overseeing Medicare and medical assistance still had an adversarial relationship with doctors and hospitals. The mission was to avoid delays in treatment and delays in discharge from the hospital for inpatients receiving care, no matter their disease or disorder. DRGs were still the payment system. Insurance companies invested a great deal of money in performing concurrent reviews of medical records of hospitalized patients.

UM nurses monitored a patient's hospitalization to ensure that each day of a hospital stay was medically necessary, there were no barriers to treatment or barriers to the patient being discharged to home or to another facility such as a nursing home, and the patient had a good clinical outcome. Hospitals now employed their own UM nurses (many of whom were previously UR nurses) to review the medical record documentation each day during the patient's hospitalization and contact the doctor if there were any barriers to treatment or to a patient's discharge that they identified. The most common problem was lack of documentation in the medical records by the doctor to justify the medical necessity for the patient to be in the hospital on a given day.

Remember that, until this point, whether it was the UR or the UM process being followed, neither the review nurses working for the outside organization nor the nurses doing chart review inside the hospital had any contact with the patient. There were also situations in which the hospital UM nurse was responsible for contacting the insurance carrier's UM department each day and reporting what specific care was being provided to the patient in order to justify her staying in the hospital "one more day." Quality of care was getting more attention now, however, and patient safety was starting to surface. PROs in particular were monitoring care from a quality perspective, raising flags when a complication would occur that was felt to be avoidable. Such instances could result in a team of doctors and nurses coming to the hospital and conducting focused reviews of specific patient populations. There was a war continuing between payers of care and the providers of care.

In the early 1990s, this process evolved yet again. Case management was born. The definition and philosophy of case management was quite different than what had been conducted previously under the UR and UM program models. Based on the needs and values of the patient and in collaboration with all her healthcare providers, the case manager (again a role fulfilled by a nurse) linked patients with appropriate providers and resources through the continuum of health and human services and care settings while ensuring that the care provided was safe, effective, patient centered, and efficient. Finally, the patient was involved, and the nurse was involved with the patient. The role went from an adversarial one to one of collaboration. The case manager was considered a vital member of the healthcare team who was involved with the patient and performed the following tasks:

1. Addressed barriers to care by ensuring that tests happened in a timely manner.
2. Educated the patient about her disease and its treatment.
3. Arranged consultations for planning the next phase of care.
4. Ensured that the team members involved with delivering care were communicating with one another.
5. Addressed psychosocial and financial issues that might affect care or delay it.
6. Arranged home care if a patient needed additional medical care after discharge.
7. Promoted patient adherence for taking oral medications at home as prescribed, and touched base with the patient after discharge with the goal of preventing the patient from an unplanned readmission to the hospital **(TABLE 2-1)**.

A particular focus was initially on patients with medical disorders who needed to be managed in a less expensive healthcare environment—either in nursing homes, in rehab centers, or at home with nurses or aides. The greatest focus of case management was on patients with chronic illnesses (diabetes, heart disease, etc.) or those with very serious illnesses (organ transplant, cancer).

TABLE 2-1 History of Nurse Navigation

Time Period	Method Used	Relationship	Treatment Setting	Timing
1970: UR	Monitor use and delivery of services	Adversarial	Inpatient	Retrospective chart review
1980: UM	Evaluate appropriateness, medical need, efficiency	Adversarial	Inpatient	Concurrent chart review
1990: Case management	Assess, plan, implement, coordinate, monitor, evaluate	Collaborative	Involved in patient care	Hands-on care
1990: Patient navigation	Identify, reduce barriers to access care, diagnose, prescribe	Collaborative	Underserved patients	Community outreach
2000: Patient navigation	Identify, reduce barriers to access care, diagnose, prescribe	Clinical collaborative	Across continuum of care, hands-on	Hands-on care and coordination of care

The healthcare system was no longer focusing only on charts and dollars but was focusing on the patient. Granted, having the patient's hospitalization not exceed the DRG limit was important, but greater emphasis was placed on improving efficiency in the care delivery process, engaging patients in their care, and carrying the management of their care into the outpatient setting. There are even some who would say that case management and patient navigation are the same.

As time progressed, more and more care became outpatient based, which was somewhat better reimbursed and less expensive than inpatient hospitalization. The focus now needed to change once again in how care was managed and monitored. As you're no doubt aware, when a patient is in an inpatient bed today, that person is very sick. Although UM programs are still in operation, justifying medical necessity for the patient staying in the hospital is rarely an issue today. And though more and more care is delivered in a more appropriate healthcare setting, it remains expensive—that's why the U.S. Federal government and managed care organizations are continuing to look at alternative ways of delivering and paying for health care.

▶ History of Patient (Lay) Navigation

When UM was established, attention was being paid to issues associated with access to care. Dr. Harold Freeman, a breast surgeon at Harlem Hospital, coined the term *patient navigation*[1,2] and brought to the attention of healthcare professionals some important information that once again changed how the delivery of healthcare services, especially those for cancer care, would be conducted. The central issue that Freeman identified and championed was that patients face a variety of barriers to standard cancer care (which includes prevention information, screening, diagnosis, treatment, and follow-up care) that inhibit timely access to healthcare services. These barriers include fragmentation of healthcare services; lack of health insurance or being underinsured; provider- and patient-related education barriers; communication barriers, particularly for patients whose first language is not English; inadequate transportation to medical appointments; and missed appointments due to travel, child care, or employment. Freeman also pointed out that health disparities arise when the delivery system does not provide access to timely, standard cancer care to everyone who needs it.[1,2] This was particularly evident among racial and ethnic minorities, people of low socioeconomic status, residents of rural areas, and members of other underserved populations.

At Harlem Hospital, Freeman implemented patient navigation to address this health disparity issue. This greatly broadened the spectrum of care. Until then, the focus had been on patients who were already familiar and "in" the healthcare model, had insurance coverage of some kind, and were undergoing treatment for a disease or disorder that had already been diagnosed. With patient navigators, the focus would begin much sooner: with routine screening. In the case of breast centers, that meant mammography screening. Navigators were responsible for educating the community about breast cancer and recruiting patients to come to the mammography facility for screening and, if needed, diagnostic evaluation.

The goal of patient navigation according to Freeman (and later adopted by the National Cancer Institute[3]) is to facilitate timely access to quality, standard cancer care in a culturally sensitive manner for all patients. Examples of navigation services include facilitating communication and information exchange for patients with a limited understanding of the English language; coordinating care among medical service providers; and arranging for financial support, transportation, and child care services. Navigators under this model could be community laypersons or healthcare professionals. Patient navigation was to span the period from cancer detection procedures (i.e., cancer screening tests) through cancer diagnostic tests and completion of treatment. This, of course, wasn't just an issue isolated to Harlem Hospital. The Institute of Medicine (IOM) report, *Care without Coverage: Too Little Too Late*,[4] states that uninsured patients get about one-half the health care of insured patients and consequently die sooner than insured patients, largely because of delayed diagnosis. Another IOM report, *Ensuring Quality Cancer Care*,[5] cites concerns about lapses in care that can lower the chances of receiving the standard of care and compromise the quality of life and survival of cancer patients.

With the transference of care from an inpatient to an outpatient setting, and managed care dictating where patients can have their treatment, more and more of the burden of keeping the schedule straight, understanding the sequence of care and treatment, and figuring out how to go from step 1 to step 2 rests with the patient. Whether the patient has cultural barriers, financial barriers, or racial barriers, the healthcare system has become incredibly complex. For someone newly diagnosed with cancer, figuring out what happens next, what to expect, and how to ensure getting appropriate care is overwhelming without help. Patients and their families are so scared and shocked by the diagnosis that navigating through decision making about treatment options as well as actually receiving the multimodality treatment in a reasonably smooth way is considered nearly impossible. In the early 2000s, the patient navigator role was expanded to encompass all patients and not just those who fit a specific underserved definition. This doesn't mean that it has only been in the last few years that cancer patients have had someone to help them along this journey. Technically, everyone involved in a cancer patient's care and treatment has always had some role in navigating the patient along the decision-making and treatment pathway, but this process was fragmented and no one had no way to assess its effectiveness. In the past, each healthcare provider focused on his or her specific portion of care, not necessarily looking across the continuum of care. Offering designated patient navigators has become popular in the last decade, and it has been particularly so in breast centers for more than two decades, primarily because it is a high-volume diagnosis nationally and there are advocacy organizations that have been providing grants to pay for navigators placed in many breast centers nationally.

A strong focus remains on addressing the needs of the underserved, recognizing that their need for patient navigation is the highest among all populations. The President's Cancer Panel (2001)[6] reported on barriers, including system barriers (fragmentation of care), financial barriers (lack of insurance or being underinsured), physical barriers (excessive distance from treatment facilities), information and education barriers (both provider- and patient-related), and the issues of culture and bias. Other barriers that were identified include insufficient, culturally sensitive information and educational materials for cancer patients and their families; inadequate transportation assistance to get to medical appointments; missed appointments due to travel or child care barriers; patients' fiscal inability to take time off from work for screening and wellness care; and failure of providers to obtain patients' medical tests or laboratory results in a timely fashion. Cultural and language barriers usually affect members of underserved populations. The cumulative effect of these barriers is unequal delivery of cancer prevention services and delays in detection, diagnosis, and quality treatment of cancers. Many racial and ethnic minorities, people of low socioeconomic status, residents of rural areas, and other underserved populations facing such barriers give up out of frustration or misunderstanding and drop out of cancer care services.

Patient (lay) navigators in a cancer center may function similarly to a case worker, helping to shepherd underserved individuals for cancer screening or, if the individuals are symptomatic, for diagnostic evaluation, and education about cancer and how to reduce the risk of getting cancer in the future. This navigator may remain involved through the patient's diagnosis or treatment, or the navigator might transition the patient to another navigator whose focus is on the diagnosis portion or treatment portion of cancer care. Some institutions do both types of navigation—pre-diagnosis and post-diagnosis. These functions are rarely done by the same person, with one being based in a community setting and filling a liaison role with the cancer center, and the other being physically based at the cancer center. Some navigation models have both patient (lay) navigators and nurse navigators working together or as a tandem team too. Remember that a patient (lay) navigator doesn't have a medical license to perform the same level of clinical support and education that a nurse navigator does, so patient and nurse navigators should not be viewed as interchangeable. Also, we always want nurses to be working to their highest level of licensure too, so having nurse navigators perform clerical tasks, which are a large part of a patient (lay) navigator's role, would not be recommended or cost efficient.

In April 2008, C-Change, a national cancer coalition comprising key national leaders from the government, business, and nonprofit sectors, hosted an educational briefing for members of Congress at the U.S. capital. The vision and mission of C-Change was to eliminate cancer as a public health problem as soon as possible by leveraging the expertise and resources of its members. The organization worked to accelerate cancer research; improve timely access to the full continuum of quality cancer care services; and support state, tribe, and territory comprehensive cancer control efforts.[7] The Cancer Patient Navigation Act was discussed. At this historic meeting, which I attended, cancer patient navigation was discussed at length, as was its importance in ensuring that cancer patients receive coordinated and high-quality, patient-focused care. Patient navigation was referred to as the individualized assistance offered to patients, families, and caregivers to help overcome healthcare system barriers and to facilitate timely access to quality medical and psychosocial care from pre-diagnosis through all the phases of the cancer experience. Navigators guide a patient through the physical, emotional, and financial challenges that come with a cancer diagnosis.[8] The Cancer Navigation Act, signed into law in June 2005, proposed spending $25 million over 5 years for demonstration projects that provide navigator services to improve health outcomes. In fiscal year (FY) 2009, C-Change and other cancer leaders asked Congress for the $25 million needed to fund the act fully.

Unfortunately, C-Change closed its doors a few years later, but the work in the navigation space continued in the hands of other active organizations. Beginning in 2009, the Academy of Oncology Nurse & Patient Navigators (AONN+) was founded and has become the only national nonprofit organization dedicated to the profession of both ONNs and patient navigators. The American Cancer Society has also invested in navigation. In recent years, it decided to invite organizations that are involved or strongly interested in the work being done within the field of oncology navigation to form the National Navigation Roundtable Network (NNRT), holding national forums and monthly conference calls to continue interactive discussions among these organizations so that knowledge is shared and the field of oncology navigation is advanced.[9] AONN+ is an active member of NNRT.

▶ History of Accreditation Requirements and Standards That Focus on Oncology Navigation

I mentioned in Chapter 1 that I would be telling you more about the Commission on Cancer (CoC). The CoC serves as the accrediting body of the American College of Surgeons for cancer centers and cancer programs to be officially accredited. They recognized the value of oncology navigation and created specific standards requiring that quality cancer care is being delivered to cancer patients. It included the importance of conducting community outreach and community needs assessments

(CNAs), identifying and eliminating barriers to care, and providing individual navigation to each cancer patient. Community outreach focuses on going into local communities served by the cancer center so that consumers can be educated, with a special focus on the underserved. In order to know that the cancer facility was aware of the need within the community it serves, the standards required that a formal needs assessment be performed every 3 years, which meant taking a serious look at the incidence of cancer in the community; what stages of disease each type of cancer was being diagnosed; other key information such as race, ethnicity, age, payer, and zip codes; and what types of myths or misinformation might exist among these residents that is preventing them from seeking screening or actual cancer care at the cancer facility being surveyed. Part of the assessment needed to include what barriers existed in the community that prevented consumers from gaining awareness, participating in early detection, practicing healthy lifestyle behaviors to reduce risk, and getting diagnosed at early stages. Such needs assessments were similar to those conducted in the early 1990s by Dr. Freeman in Harlem when he was trying to determine how to reduce mortality among local residents who were being diagnosed with breast cancer at a later stage, what is sometimes referred to as "late stage neglected breast cancer." By combining the needs assessment findings and using those results as part of the research information learned, cancer centers could begin a more pragmatic approach to developing and implementing a navigation program. Note I didn't say that the cancer center was to start hiring navigators. The standard doesn't state this either.

The standards associated with navigation, along with other standards such as survivorship care, went through an onerous and thoughtful review process by the Clinical Services Revision Workgroup of the CoC in 2018 and 2019. It was an arduous task and was referred to as the CoC Standards Revision Project. I was fortunate to serve on the Clinical Services Revision Workgroup representing AONN+, which became the fifty-third member of the CoC several years ago. I serve as the fellow representing AONN+, so you can consider me your voice within the CoC, if you choose to join me and become an AONN+ member.

The CoC standards focus on the cancer center having an effective navigation program. The goal of the Standards Revision Project was to ensure that each standard results in the improvement of patient care. Therefore, each standard must meet defined principles, be backed up by evidence-based research information, and identify new ways to confirm compliance (especially when a physician surveyor is onsite conducting the triannual review). Steps were also taken to incorporate operative standards for cancer surgery, which were new for the CoC to measure. All of the revisions must be clearly interpretable and should be objectively verifiable by experienced physician surveyors. Many other standards were also revised, but for the purposes of this discussion, I want to bring to your attention that navigation standards exist and that you should be a key individual who has the opportunity to meet the physician reviewer (previously known as the physician surveyor) when he or she comes to your facility. You also will be one of the individuals providing data prior to the survey for electronic review several months ahead of the scheduled survey site visit. I would be remiss if I didn't include for you the Survivorship Standard as well because it too is a standard with which you will be personally involved. This standard was difficult to achieve due to its prior mandate of providing each cancer patient a treatment summary and survivorship care plan (SCP). You will see that the Clinical Services Revision Workgroup worked hard on this standard to learn what was needed, which goes beyond a patient receiving a document. The revised standards are to be implemented in 2020, with their release date announced to cancer centers in September 2019. The revised standards are listed below for you to get a preview of what is to come; also recorded for your review are the previous versions of these standards from 2012 and 2016 when they were originally written and subsequently revised.[10]

▶ Continuum of Care Services Standards from the CoC Standards Manual of 2016

The Continuum of Care Services Standards are found in Section 3.

Standard 3.1: Patient Navigation Process (2012)

A patient navigation process, driven by a CNA, is established to address healthcare disparities and barriers to care for patients. Resources to address identified barriers may be provided either onsite or by referral to community-based or national organizations. The navigation process is evaluated, documented, and reported to the cancer committee annually. The patient navigation process is modified or enhanced each year to address additional barriers identified by the CNA.

Definition and Requirements

Patient navigation in cancer care refers to individualized assistance offered to patients, families, and caregivers to help overcome healthcare system barriers and facilitate timely access to quality medical and psychosocial care and can occur from prior to a cancer diagnosis through all phases of the cancer experience. The navigation services implemented depend on the particular type, severity, and/or complexity of the identified barriers.

Prior to establishing the navigation process, the cancer committee conducts a CNA at least once during the 3-year survey cycle to identify: the needs of the population served, potential to improve cancer health disparities, and gaps in resources. The results from this CNA can serve as the building blocks for program development, implementation, and evaluation. The cancer committee may delegate the responsibility for the CNA and program implementation to a specified individual, subcommittee, or department. The CNA results are documented in the cancer committee minutes.

The CNA can be used to guide the initiatives planned to comply with the community outreach standards and/or the psychosocial services eligibility criteria. The completion of the CNA does not fulfill the requirement of the CoC, however. This information needs to be analyzed and is used to promote awareness, to achieve early detection of cancers and be measurable, looking at statistics associated with cancer incidence and stages of these cancers on the basis of the findings within the CNA and then comparing those statistics to the outcomes achieved after the necessary interventions were performed.

The cancer committee, or a responsible designee, selects appropriate tools to perform the CNA. The cancer committee evaluates and reports on the navigation process annually. The evaluation and report include, but are not limited to, the following:

- Health disparities identified
- Description of the navigation process
- Population(s) served and barriers identified by the CNA
- Documentation of activities and metrics (outcomes/outputs)
- Areas for QI, enhancement, and future directions

Measuring Compliance Rating

(1) **Compliance:** The program fulfills the following criteria:

1. Conducts a CNA at least once during the 3-year survey cycle to address healthcare disparities and barriers to care for patients.
2. Establishes a patient navigation process and identifies resources to address barriers that are provided either onsite or by referral to community-based or national organizations.
3. Assesses each year barriers to care, the navigation process is evaluated and documented, and the findings are reported to the cancer committee.
4. The patient navigation process is modified or enhanced each year to address additional barriers identified by the CNA.

Noncompliance: The program does not fulfill one or more of the following criteria:

1. Conducts a CNA at least once during the 3-year survey cycle to address healthcare disparities and barriers to care for patients.
2. Establishes a patient navigation process and identifies resources to address barriers that are provided either onsite or by referral to community-based or national organizations.
3. Assesses each year barriers to care, the navigation process is evaluated and documented, and the findings are reported to the cancer committee.
4. The patient navigation process is modified or enhanced each year to address additional barriers identified by the CNA.

Standard 3.3: Survivorship Care Plan (2012)

The cancer committee develops and implements a process to disseminate a comprehensive care summary and follow-up plan to patients with cancer who are completing cancer treatment. The process is monitored, evaluated, and presented at least annually to the cancer committee and documented in the minutes.

Definitions and Requirements

The IOM and National Research Council 2005 report, *From Cancer Patient to Cancer Survivor: Lost in Transition,* recommends that patients with cancer who are completing the first of course treatment be "provided with a comprehensive care summary and follow-up plan that is clearly and effectively explained." The recommendation suggested that these plans would help cancer survivors who may otherwise get lost in the transitions from the care they received during treatment through the phases of their life or stages of their disease course. The purpose of this standard is to have cancer programs develop and implement a process to monitor the dissemination of a SCP as part of the standard care of patients with cancer. The process is implemented, monitored, evaluated, and presented annually to the cancer committee. The presentation is documented in the minutes.

The written or electronic SCP contains a record of care received, important disease characteristics, and a follow-up care plan incorporating available and recognized evidence-based standards of care, when available. The minimum care plan standards are included in "Fact Sheet: Cancer Survivorship Care Planning" from the IOM.

Additional resources are available to assist programs with the development of these tools, including care planning templates. Care planning templates are available from, for example, the American Society of Clinical Oncology, National Coalition for Cancer Survivorship, and Lance Armstrong Foundation.

Compliance Measurement Rating

Ten percent, initially, then 25% of patients meeting the criteria are to receive an SCP during a face-to-face consultation with an oncology provider who was directly involved in their treatment. Then it was raised to 50%, which was quite difficult for cancer centers to achieve.

Implementation of the standard and required percentage of SCPs provided must follow the schedule as outlined:

- January 1, 2015–December 31, 2015: Implement process to provide SCPs to ≥10% of eligible patients who have completed treatment.
- End of 2016: Provide SCPs to ≥25% of eligible patients who have completed treatment.
- End of 2017: Provide SCPs to ≥50% of eligible patients who have completed treatment.
- End of 2018 onward: Provide SCPs to ≥75% of eligible patients who have completed treatment.

The 2018 requirement was not achievable for most cancer centers, so it was reduced and maintained at the 2017 level, being >50%. However, even this was difficult for many.

Standard 3.1: Patient Navigation Process (2016)

A patient navigation process, driven by a triennial CNA, is established to address healthcare disparities and barriers to cancer care. Resources to address identified barriers may be provided either onsite or by referral.

Definition and Requirements

Patient navigation in cancer care refers to specialized assistance for the community, patients, families, and caregivers to assist in overcoming barriers to receiving care and facilitating timely access to clinical services and resources. Navigation processes encompass pre-diagnosis through all phases of the cancer experience. The navigation services implemented depend on the particular type, severity, and/or complexity of the identified barriers. Prior to establishing the navigation process, the cancer committee must conduct a CNA at least once every 3 years during the 3-year accreditation cycle. The cancer committee defines the scope, selects appropriate tools to perform the CNA, and is involved in the assessment and evaluation of results. Local, county, and state cancer-related information may be utilized in obtaining data. The cancer committee may work with outreach and/or marketing departments as well as community-based organizations outside the facility to accomplish a robust CNA.

The CNA must define/identify the following:

- The cancer program's community and local patient population
- Health disparities (numerous factors can contribute to disparities in cancer incidence and death such as race, ethnicity, gender, underserved groups, and socioeconomic status)
- Barriers to care, which may include patient-centered, provider-centered, or health system–centered barriers
- Resources available to overcome barriers onsite or by formal referral
- Gaps in the availability of resources to overcome barriers

The results from the CNA serve as the building blocks for navigation process development, implementation, and evaluation. Data and results of the CNA are presented to the cancer committee and documented in the cancer committee minutes. As part of establishing the appropriate patient navigation to address the results of the CNA, the cancer committee will construct a report including, but not limited to, the following:

- Population(s) to be served that were identified by the CNA
- Health disparities and barriers identified by the CNA
- Description of the navigation process to overcome barriers
- Documentation of activities and outcomes of the navigation process
- Areas for improvement, enhancement, and future directions

To improve the quality of patient navigation continually, a new barrier should be addressed each calendar year. However, programs are allowed to address the same barrier or disparity for more than one year as long as the cancer committee determines that addressing the barrier is the most important concern and an ongoing need for its community. Documentation should demonstrate the efforts put forth over the year and that there is an ongoing need to continue addressing the barrier in an attempt to make more significant progress to address the barrier.

The completion of the CNA does not fulfill the requirement for Standard 4.7: Studies of Quality. *This standard does not require the hiring of a patient navigator but rather focuses on the processes to understand health disparity populations and rectify barriers to care.*

Standard 3.3: Survivorship Care Plan (2016)

The cancer committee develops and implements a process to disseminate a treatment summary and follow-up plan to patients who have completed cancer treatment. The process is monitored and evaluated annually by the cancer committee.

Definition and Requirements

The IOM report *From Cancer Patient to Cancer Survivor*[4] outlines the importance of providing cancer survivors with a comprehensive treatment summary and follow-up plan (i.e., SCP) that reflects the treatment they received and addresses post-treatment needs and follow-up care to improve health and quality of life.

The SCP summarizes and communicates what transpired during active cancer treatment, provides recommendations for follow-up care and surveillance testing/ examinations, offers referrals for support services that the patient may need going forward, and lists other information pertinent to the survivor's short- and long-term survivorship care.

The American Society of Clinical Oncology (ASCO) has defined the minimum data elements to be included in a treatment summary and SCP. This core set of data elements and templates is available on the ASCO website (www.asco.org). At a minimum, all SCPs must include ASCO's recommended elements describing treatment summary and a follow-up care plan to meet compliance for this standard. Additional resources to assist with the development of SCPs are available through the National Coalition for Cancer Survivorship, Journey Forward, American Cancer Society, and LIVESTRONG Foundation.

Process Requirements

Cancer programs must develop and implement processes to monitor the formation and dissemination of an SCP for analytic cases with Stage I, II, or III cancers that are treated with curative intent for initial cancer occurrence and who have completed active therapy.

Within the SCP processes are policies and procedures identifying the appropriate healthcare provider(s) from patients' oncology care team who will be responsible for approving and discussing the SCP. Providers who are part of the patient's care team that are appropriate under the standard to deliver the SCP include:

- Physicians
- Registered nurses
- Advanced practice nurses
- Nurse practitioners
- Physician assistants
- Credentialed clinical navigators (does not include lay navigators)

The printed or electronic SCP must contain input from the principal physician and oncology care team who coordinated the oncology treatment for the patient, as well as input from the patient's other care providers (outside treatment information), if applicable. If two separate facilities are providing treatment, both facilities collaborate to complete and provide the SCP. In all cases, programs, hospitals, and physician offices should work together to provide the information necessary for completion of an SCP that contains all required elements.

The SCP is given to and discussed with the patient upon completion of active, curative treatment and recorded in the patient medical record. The timing of delivery of the SCP is within 1 year of the diagnosis of cancer and no later than 6 months after completion of adjuvant therapy (other than long-term hormonal therapy). The "1 year from diagnosis" requirement to have an SCP delivered is extended to 18 months for patients receiving long-term hormonal therapy. Providing the SCP by mail, electronically, or through a patient portal without discussion with the patient does not meet the standard.

Compliance Rating Measurement

Fifty percent of patients who meet the criteria are to have received an SCP face-to-face with an oncology provider who was directly involved in their treatment.

▶ What Does This Mean for an ONN?

It takes more than hiring you as an ONN to truly have an effective navigation program. You are a key component of it, but there is much more. You are key to an effective and innovative cancer survivorship program too.

Meeting these past standards was not easy and required a lot of work and a great deal of documentation. (Remember what we learned in nursing school—if it isn't documented, then it wasn't done.) There is also a standard for performing a distress measurement of each cancer patient at a pivotal visit. I decided not to include that standard in this section because, frankly, you may not be the person responsible for performing that task. If you are, however, then visit the reference document which can be accessed at https://www.facs.org/quality-programs/cancer/coc/standards, where you can read the details of Standard 3.2. In the revised standards that go into effect from January 2020, it is now a part of section 5, within Standard 5.3: Psychosocial Distress Screening.[10]

Standard 3.3: Survivorship Care Plan has been the hardest for cancer centers to achieve. It doesn't matter if they are large or small, have expertise in creating SCPs or not, it is a very costly standard to meet. There also wasn't enough evidence-based research conducted prior to its original implementation to ensure that a patient receiving such a document experienced better clinical outcomes. For example, did the patient follow the recommendations for adopting healthier lifestyle habits that were discussed with him? Did he quit smoking as recommended? Did another patient follow up at the right intervals and get her subsequent cancer screenings performed? Is she still adhering to the chronic medications she is to be taking to prevent recurrence or has she arbitrarily stopped taking them due to side effects that are affecting her quality of life? You can see why there was a lot of discussion about this specific standard and how there may be formidable measures taken to alter its expectations and intentions so that it measured what we needed it to measure. I admit I was a squeaky wheel regarding this standard in its current form. The best intentions were certainly the driving force for its development, and it undoubtedly seemed logical at the time to create it. Now with more experience and more time, it has become clear that the standard was measuring what was really important.

Below are revised Standards 8.1 and 8.3 to be implemented in 2020. Note first that the numbers for these standards have changed too as some standards were incorporated into other established standards or developed into new standards. Take a look at this chart to see what the "old" standard numbers were and what they have now become. This will help you as you continue to read the revised standards information below.

Commission on Cancer Standards Closely Aligned with Oncology Navigation	
Old Version of Standard (2016)	**New Version of Standard (Effective Jan 2020)**
3.1 Patient Navigation Process	8.1 Addressing Barriers to Care
3.2 Psychosocial Distress Screening	5.3 Psychosocial Distress Screening
3.3 Survivorship Care Plan	4.8 Survivorship Program
4.1 Cancer Prevention Program	8.2 Cancer Prevention Event
4.2 Cancer Screening Program	8.3 Cancer Screening Event

The revised standards covering the new content and requirements of Standard 3.1 are now found in Section 8, entitled Education: Professional and Community Outreach. There are also title changes. Standard 8.1 is Addressing Barriers to Care. Standard 8.2 is Cancer Prevention Event. Standard 8.3 is Cancer Screening Event. Previously Cancer Prevention and Screening Event standards were in Standards 4.1 and 4.2. The revised standards for 3.3, the standard associated with survivorship, can now be found in Standard 4.9. Please note that the title for the survivorship standard also changed, and quite significantly. It was 3.3: Survivorship Care Plan, and now it is 4.9: Survivorship Care Program. There may be additional minor changes made to these and possibly other standards. Visit the CoC's website to see what additional information or edits were performed. The information provided here is up-to-date as of August 20, 2019, which was a month after the CoC held its final meeting to review all of the standards and approve them. I felt fortunate, as a representative of AONN+, to be able to review those standards that are tied to clinical services.

Standard 8.1: Addressing Barriers to Care Beginning January 2020

This is the final draft of the standard as of August 20, 2019, a month after the CoC meeting to finalize all the revisions made to all the standards.

Definition and Requirements

Patient navigation in cancer care is specialized assistance for the community, patients, families, and caregivers to assist in overcoming barriers to receiving care and facilitating timely access to clinical services and resources.

Navigation Processes. Navigation processes encompass pre-diagnosis through all phases of the cancer experience. The navigation services implemented depend on the particular type, severity, and/or complexity of the identified barriers. Each calendar year, the cancer committee identifies at least one patient, system, or provider-based barrier to accessing health and/or psychosocial care that its patients with cancer are facing and develops and implements a plan to address the barrier.

Cancer Barriers Analysis. The cancer committee reviews and analyzes the strengths and barriers of the cancer program. Resources for identifying strengths and barriers may include, but are not limited to:

- Cancer Quality Improvement Program (CQIP) reports
- Cancer patient satisfaction surveys
- Patient focus groups
- Use of state cancer registry data compared to your cancer center data
  - Are you treating the main cancers that occur in your area?
  - Are you reaching vulnerable populations?
- Population health resources from public health work done locally and regionally
- CNA
- Analysis of unique features of your institution and/or state (e.g., affordable or adequate lodging for patients receiving care at a rural facility)

Identification of Barriers. Each calendar year, the cancer committee identifies barriers that are specific to the cancer program and chooses one to focus on for the upcoming year. Examples include, but are not limited to:

- Gaps in community resources
- Identified populations in need
- Uninsured or underinsured
- Healthcare provider shortages

Each calendar year, the cancer committee minutes document a report that includes all required elements:

- What barrier was chosen
- What resources/processes were utilized to identify and address this barrier
- Metrics related to outcomes of reducing the chosen barrier

Documentation

Submitted with pre-review questionnaire:

- Cancer committee minutes documenting the required report to the cancer committee.
  Each calendar year, the program fulfills the compliance criteria:
  1. The cancer committee identifies at least one barrier to focus on for the year and identifies resources and processes to address the barrier.
  2. At the end of the year, the cancer committee evaluates the resources and processes adopted to address the barrier to care and identifies strengths and areas for improvement.
  3. The cancer committee minutes include all required elements.

Standard 4.9: Survivorship Program Beginning January 2020

This is the final draft of the standard as of July 9, 2019, prior to the CoC meeting to finalize all the revisions made to all the standards.

Definition and Requirements

The cancer committee oversees the development and implementation of a survivorship program directed at meeting the needs of cancer patients treated with curative intent.

Survivorship Program Team. The cancer committee appoints a coordinator of the survivorship program per the requirements in Standard 2.1: Cancer Committee. The survivorship program coordinator develops a survivorship program team. Suggested members include physicians, advanced practice providers, nurses, social workers, nutritionists, physical therapists, and other allied health professionals. The survivorship program team determines a list of services and programs, offered onsite or by referral, that address the needs of cancer survivors. The team formally documents a minimum of three services offered each year. Services may be continued year-to-year, but it is expected that cancer programs will strive to enhance existing services over time and develop new services.

Each year, the survivorship program coordinator gives a report, and the cancer committee reviews the activities of the survivorship program. The report includes:

- An estimate of the number of cancer patients who participated in three identified services to assist with identification of which programs were effective
- Identification of the resources needed to improve the programs if barriers were encountered

Survivorship Program Services. Services utilized by the survivorship program may include, but are not limited to:

- Treatment summaries and SCPs
- Screening programs for cancer recurrence
- Screening for new cancers
- Seminars for survivors
- Physical therapy
- Nutritional services
- Psychological support and psychiatric services
- Support groups and services
- Formalized referrals to experts in cardiology, pulmonary services, sexual dysfunction, and fertility counseling
- Financial support services
- Fitness programs

Treatment Summaries and SCPs. The CoC recommends that patients receive and encourages patients to receive a treatment summary and SCP, but delivery of such plans is not a required component of this standard anymore. Delivery of

SCPs may be utilized as one of the services offered to survivors to meet the requirements of this standard. If so, then the program defines the population to receive care plans.

Documentation

Submitted with pre-review questionnaire:

- Policy and procedure defining the survivorship program requirements
- Cancer committee minutes that document the required yearly evaluation of the survivorship program.

Measure of Compliance

Each calendar year, the program fulfills all of the following compliance criteria:

1. The cancer committee identifies a survivorship program team, including its designated coordinator and members.
2. The survivorship program is monitored and evaluated. A report is given to the cancer committee, contains all required elements, and is documented in the cancer committee minutes.

You as an ONN should be, and I hope will be, directly involved in fulfilling these two specific standards in the cancer facility where you are or will be working. As a matter of fact, you could even become the survivorship care program coordinator for your institution!

As mentioned earlier, there are also revised standards for cancer prevention and community outreach, which are the other two standards that make up Chapter 8: Education: Professional and Community Outreach. I didn't want to overwhelm you with too much, however, because a different navigator, such as a patient lay navigator, may be more involved with community outreach programs and promoting cancer screenings.

You may already be familiar with the oncology nursing credentials standard. It is now Standard 4.2. I am thrilled to tell you that once AONN+ achieves its accreditation status for our ONN certification program, I hope that the credentials ONN-CG (Certified General) (which you may be able to add after your name in the future) will be incorporated into this standard as well. Only certification programs that are accredited are to be recognized by the CoC.

If you are still in the interviewing process, inquire of those interviewing you how well the institution performed during its last triannual survey and what year it was performed. This will help you in knowing what additional work will be needed to fulfill the new standards and maintain compliance with them. If your cancer center is not accredited by the CoC, try to find out why. It is by no means a requirement to be accredited, but patients can feel a higher level of confidence if they are receiving their care at a CoC-accredited facility.

Accreditation programs exist specifically for two subspecialties: breast centers and rectal cancer centers. These two accreditation programs are also not required. The accreditation process is very similar to the overall cancer center accreditation process except that it is specific for patients who have breast cancer or rectal cancer; it includes screening, early detection, diagnosis, treatment, and survivorship/end of life. These two diagnostic categories were chosen because (1) the number of breast cancer patients is very large, and (2) rectal cancer has been identified as a type of cancer that is not consistently treated according to National Comprehensive Cancer Network (NCCN) treatment guidelines. The CoC felt a closer focus was needed, which makes sense.

Will other subspecialty cancer categories be identified? That isn't known yet. However, the CoC, under the direction of the American College of Surgeons, has begun to implement standards that are specific to surgical management.[10]

In Chapter 3, we are going to dig more deeply into formal roles and responsibilities, the various models of navigation, and something you may not know a lot about yet but should—the world of oncopolitics.

▶ Summary

In this chapter, we have started to discuss oncology nurse navigation, beginning with the history of navigation. As I mentioned, if you don't know where your role came from, then it may be hard to see where you are going. The history that I provided also included the history of patient lay navigation. Keep in mind that you may have an opportunity to work alongside a patient lay navigator, a social worker who is performing some navigation functions, or a financial navigator too. The functions, roles, and expectations of an ONN were also reviewed, including what patients believe their ONN can do to help them.

Another important component of this chapter was a discussion about what cancer center leadership might expect of you as an ONN. It is so important that everyone communicates and that there is no confusion or miscommunication about your roles, responsibilities, goals, and objectives as an ONN.

Last, I provided detailed information about how the CoC has incorporated into its standards the importance of institutions having a navigation program as well as a survivorship care program. These standards, first written in 2012, and have evolved, with the greatest evolution to take place at the beginning of 2020. Your role with both navigation and survivorship will have a great impact, and I hope you have a voice at the table when planning for a CoC triannual accreditation process, and I hope that you can be available for questions when the physician reviewer is onsite at your cancer facility.

References

1. Shockney L. *Becoming a Breast Cancer Nurse Navigator.* Boston, MA: Jones & Bartlett Publishers, 2011.
2. Harold P. Freeman Institute for Patient Navigation. *Fact Sheet* [Web page]. New York, NY: The Institute, 2009. http://www.hpfreemanpni.org. Accessed May 3, 2019.
3. Patient Navigation Research Program, Center to Reduce Cancer Health Disparities, National Cancer Institute. *PNRP Brochure.* Rockville, MD: National Cancer Institute, 2009. http://crchd .cancer.gov/attachments/pnrp_brochure.pdf. Accessed May 2, 2019.
4. Institute of Medicine. *Care without Coverage: Too Little, Too Late.* Washington, DC: National Academy Press. http://www.iom.edu/en/Reports/2003/Care-Without-Coverage-Too-Little-Too -Late.aspx. Accessed May 2, 2019.
5. Institute of Medicine. *Ensuring Quality Cancer Care.* Washington, DC: National Academy Press. http://www.iom.edu/en/Reports/2003/Ensuring-Quality-Cancer-Care.aspx. Accessed May 2, 2019.

6. National Cancer Institute, Division of Extramural Activities. President's Cancer Panel Annual Report for 2000–2001 with Video. http://deainfo.nci.nih.gov/advisory/pcp/video-report.htm. Accessed May 2, 2019.

7. C-Change. About C-Change. http://www.c-changetogether.org/about_ndc/default.asp. Accessed November 5, 2009.

8. Bio-Medicine. Support for Patient Navigation Services to Help Cancer Patients. http://www.bio-medicine.org/medicine-news-1/Support-for-Patient-Navigation-Services-to-Help-Cancer-Patients-17607-1. Accessed May 2, 2019.

9. National Navigation Roundtable Network. https://navigationroundtable.org. Accessed May 2, 2019.

10. Commission on Cancer website. https://www.facs.org/quality-programs/cancer/coc/standards. Accessed May 5, 2019.

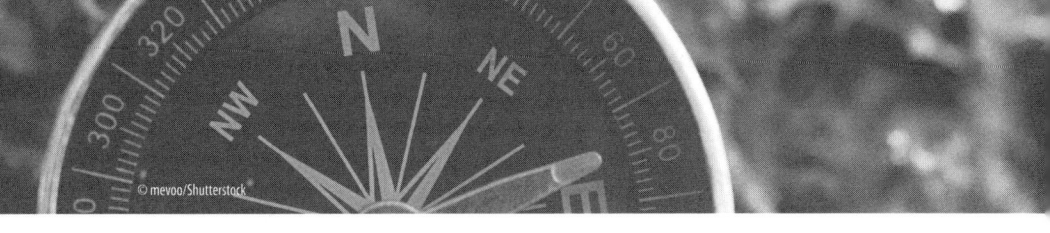

CHAPTER 3

Roles, Responsibilities, Models of Navigation, and Oncopolitics

Now it is time to start discussing what your formal roles and responsibilities are, as well as various models of navigation programs that can serve as a starting point for you and your manager to begin using as a template for designing what your navigation duties will be. I would be remiss if I didn't include the pitfalls that can almost always become barriers to developing and implementing a navigation program, as well as to your being successful as an oncology nurse navigator (ONN) from the very start.

▶ Roles and Responsibilities of an ONN Based on Professional Standards

I provided you information Chapters 1 and 2 that described from the patient's viewpoint what your roles and responsibilities might be. I included in that information also what expectations patients and your own cancer center leadership may have of you too. Now let's talk about what your roles and functions are based on thoughtful analysis, years of experience, and careful study that has been conducted by the Academy of Oncology Nurse & Patient Navigators (AONN+) over the last 10 years.[1]

▶ Overview of Professional Roles and Responsibilities

The guiding principles of patient navigation are to ensure that quality, confidentiality, and professionalism are threaded throughout all aspects of care and programming.[4]

Inherent in the process is continuous quality care for patients, from screening through diagnosis and treatment, based on the following tenets:

- Culturally competent care
- Confidentiality
- Respect
- Compassion
- Patient safety

Common responsibilities of a nurse navigator include the following:

- Providing education and support to the patient and family
- Identifying special needs of the patient and delegating to appropriate support staff
- Enhancing understanding of treatment options available
- Facilitating patient care plan recommendations by the physician
- Connecting patient and family with community resources
- Coordinating multidisciplinary care from the time of diagnosis throughout treatment
- Improving timeliness of appointments
- Serving as a resource for the community on health issues, prevention, screening, treatment, and research

Confusion can exist about the navigator roles and responsibilities. Nurse navigators commonly spend time doing clerical tasks such as faxing documents, waiting on the phone for precertification, and scheduling appointments for patients. This time is best spent *with* patients in education, psychosocial counseling, and facilitating multidisciplinary care. On the AONN+ website, the definition of navigators describes this distinction.[1] Willis and colleagues published work about a collaborative project with national stakeholders in navigation to create a role delineation framework.[2] The final framework is composed of 12 functional domains, with differences between community health workers, patient navigators, and clinically licensed navigators described in each frame.

Skills such as advocacy, problem solving, time management, critical thinking, multitasking, collaboration, and communication were identified in the Oncology Nursing Society oncology nurse navigation role delineation study.[3] AONN+, however, has identified additional skills of leadership and systems management. Leadership skills of the nurse navigator are expressed in several publications, and the role is depicted as one that often survives in a macro-managed environment—one that needs minimal supervision. Seek and Hogle stressed this leadership skill as the navigator works through the complex healthcare system to coordinate optimal care.[4] Blaseg describes this set of skills (problem solving, time management, critical thinking, working well independently) as a desired quality for a nurse navigator—one who can make decisions and work independently within the bounds of the role and demonstrate personal and professional accountability with a commitment to lifelong learning.[5] According to Vargas and colleagues, ONNs remain flexible to possibilities of care.[6] Systems management is best described by Fillion and colleagues, who wrote that the workflow of nurse navigation is two-dimensional—patient-centered and health system–oriented.[7] Doll and colleagues state that nurse navigators possess oversight of the comprehensive care needs; provide education and advocacy for the patient; link the patient to networks of professional and community resources; and act as a distinct, constant contact to enhance psychosocial care.[8] An example of this systemic overview is shown in the work by Christensen and Bellomo with the navigation process that demonstrated a decrease in system time as well as a cost advantage to the healthcare system.[9]

Visit the AONN+ website (www.aonnonline.org) to read more details about roles and responsibilities. Some information is in front of the firewall and other content is behind it, reserved for members. I am confident, however, by just touching on the information provided above, you can see how vital a role you play for the patient and for the cancer center as well. It is an amazing role to serve in and one that brings new clinical and psychosocial situations to you every day.

▶ Begin Survivorship Care at the Moment of Diagnosis

What does it mean to begin survivorship care at the moment of diagnosis? Historically, the goal of cancer treatment was for the patient to complete treatment and survive it. If the patient was alive at the end of treatment, then the treatment team believed that it had been successful in saving another life from cancer. This is a very outdated way to look at clinical outcomes, with the only measure being that of mortality rates. Today patients don't want just to survive; they want to survive with good quality of life. This is a game changer. The only way to make that happen is to begin survivorship as soon as the patient's diagnosis is known.[10] This means that you, as the patient's ONN, need to gather a lot of personal information about patients and their lives.

For example, what are the patients' life goals? Where do they see themselves in 1 year, 5 years, 10 years from now? Perhaps a female patient is planning to start a family in another 1 to 2 years, before she heard she her diagnosis of cancer. If this patient has a type of cancer that has a relatively early stage, she will likely need a referral to fertility preservation experts to harvest eggs and/or create embryos, or her partner may need sperm harvested for future use. If the patient is up for a promotion at work, she may want to work as much as she can during treatment to demonstrate to her boss her true commitment to the corporation. For someone who is hoping to complete her teaching degree but has just gotten started, she may need a treatment plan that enables her to go to school during treatment with as little disruption as possible. We don't want to derail a patient's life; we want to keep them on track for what is important to them, and life goals are very important. Cancer patients should only give cancer what is needed to treat it and not let it steal away any more time than is necessary, and certainly not their life goals. Cancer doesn't deserve it. Patients should not allow cancer to get that kind of power. They need to remain on track for their life goals too.

What if your patient has advanced disease? This patient may be planning to retire in 10 years but now is diagnosed with an advanced stage of pancreatic cancer. Does this mean that you and the treatment team will tell the patient that he will work with them to achieve this life goal? We need to be optimistic for as long as it is realistic. (Remember that quote from me.) We can likely provide some clinical trial options for this patient that may extend life, but then again, maybe a clinical trial won't help him at all. In this case, you need to do a different type of interview with the patient. What you will likely learn is that the patient is aware of the gravity of his disease and doesn't want to leave his family with financial ruin. He may want to talk more about the cost of some treatment options and really weigh in what he does and doesn't want to do, always enabling him to remain the one in charge of the decision making about his treatment. This means you may need to be his advocate and serve as his voice with his family members, who might insist he try one more (very expensive) treatment, despite it having a very low probability of helping him. Or you may be speaking up for him at tumor board meetings, letting the team know what he has candidly shared with you about his wishes not to make his family bankrupt for the sake of him existing a few more months. In such a case, the patient's life goal is that he wants to leave enough money for his family to live and not put them into financial debt by taking additional treatments that will not save his life.

As you can see, at times your job is daunting. The fact is that, today, although more and more people are surviving cancer, there continue to be many who will not. The type of cancer patients you will be navigating will determine if you will have mostly survivors, a mixture of survivors and victims, or even mostly victims. No matter what your patient population is that you will support, it is an amazing role to fill on these patients' behalf.

Specific milestones are likely to come up during, let's say, 9 to 12 months of treatment that carry great importance to the patient and her family. Perhaps a daughter is marrying in 4 weeks or a grandson is graduating from high school. As part of your information gathering from the patient during that first encounter you have, you will need to inquire about these milestones too. Patients are usually so worried about dying of cancer that they will tell you these milestones don't matter anymore. But when they look back over this time in their lives, they need to be able to remember the joy they experiences at a daughter's wedding and the pride they felt watching a grandson walk across the stage to get his diploma. This is only possible by dovetailing these milestones within a treatment plan.

For example, a patient may have told the breast surgeon that she wants her mastectomy surgery right away, and he may accommodate her by scheduling her for mastectomy, sentinel node biopsy with tissue expander insertion 3 weeks from now, not yet knowing that her daughter's wedding will be taking place 8 days later. But you can intervene to educate the patient by explaining that delaying the surgery until after the wedding isn't increasing her risk of the cancer spreading and that it is important to preserve such milestones. She would look funny walking down the aisle in her mother-of-the-bride gown with Jackson Pratt drains bulging from underneath it. At the reception she would have difficulty dancing with her new tall son-in-law because she can't get her arm up and around his shoulder comfortably due to one of the drains in her axilla. And she would hope that time would go by faster so the reception would be over and she could go home and get back in bed. This certainly would not be the memories that she had originally planned to experience before she was diagnosed.

Thus, preservation of life goals and milestone moments need to be a priority. You will provide documentation in the patient's electronic medical record for the entire treatment team to see as well as verbally discuss these with each provider at the point that decisions are made about treatments and when they are to happen. Of course, you will always be focusing too on helping to ensure that the patient remains on track for receiving treatment that is in keeping with National Comprehensive Cancer Network (NCCN) treatment guidelines.[11] There are rare circumstances, however, when cancer treatment must begin immediately, within days of the diagnosis. When this does occur, life milestones are sometimes forfeited, or perhaps they can be moved to a later time if they carry great significance.

▶ How to Fit Well and Be Recognized as a Valuable Member within a Multidisciplinary Team

If you were functioning as a clinical oncology nurse (CON) with the same multidisciplinary team in which you are currently working as an ONN, then there is good news and bad news. The good news is that you know all the players, and you are well informed about how the clinic runs, who does what, and so on. You know who is challenging and who is easy to work with, and what some of the pitfalls might be. But there are challenges, too. One challenge is that the team members are accustomed to having you function as a CON. Although your role has changed or perhaps soon will, in their minds, it may not have, and you may be pulled into doing CON tasks that now are supposed to be the responsibility of another CON. There are also preconceived ideas of what an ONN is supposed to be doing, which can look totally different than the list of roles and responsibilities I have previously discussed in this chapter. Frankly, you might be seen as the new person to dump tasks on that no one else wants to do. Suddenly a bunch of clerical work appears on your desk that you didn't think would become your responsibility.

Before things get out of hand or go adrift, you need to discuss with your supervisor what your ONN job description is to entail and put it in writing. All members of the multidisciplinary team should have copies of it, and actually understand it, before you begin your new role as an ONN. Many ONNs have an accurate job description, but the tasks and functions they end up performing do not fit that job description at all. And don't be an enabler. It's so easy for a doctor to walk up to you and say, "This probably isn't your job but I need this done now and I know you will know how to do it. Do please take these papers and do this for me." Instead of agreeing, confirm what the specific need is and quickly identify in your mind who is the right person to perform this task, then tell the doctor you will work with "so and so" to get this done since this is part of so and so's responsibilities and you want to respect everyone's job boundaries. Then take the documents to that person whose job description it is to do this task and tell him or her that the doctor has requested this be done and that it be expedited. If you don't do this, it will be more and more difficult to reverse it. Stand strong!

Now I realize you may be sighing right now as you read these words. My intention is not to overwhelm you but instead to provide you with the tools, resources, and skills you need to stand tall. I also want you to be able to begin this new and wonderful role without having to be pleasing everyone constantly. Remember that your responsibilities are to support the patient. Each person has her or his own defined roles and responsibilities as to how to support the patient.

What is ideal is to make a chart of everyone's roles and responsibilities. Some charts may be simple and others more comprehensive. Request that your supervisor work on the chart with you and include everyone on the team. This allows everyone to see a clear delineation of responsibilities, with avoidance of overlap too. You will always need to be able to articulate what you do, and simply saying that you navigate patients won't suffice. It's too vague. Review again the roles and responsibilities and make sure you are clear on each one. You may be working alongside a patient lay navigator too who obviously has "navigator" in her title like you. The need becomes increasingly important to have clear delineation of responsibilities so you and the patient lay navigator know where yours begin and hers start. This is a collaborative relationship; however, it still needs to have boundaries.

It is important for you to record specifically what you do, how you do it, when it is done, where it happens, and why. Here's an example of a breast surgical consultation:

- Who—ONN
- What—arrange for patients' surgical consultation appointments
- Where—in the surgical clinic of the breast center
- When—as soon as the biopsy results confirm a diagnosis of breast cancer
- How—by calling the appointment scheduler to procure an appointment and then calling the patient to inform her of the date and educating her about what to expect at the time of this consultation with a breast surgeon
- Why—to expedite evaluation of the patient getting the treatment plan underway, to provide the patient with a point of contact to address her psychological needs, and to begin the education process overall about her treatment

▶ How Your Supervisor's Role Affects Your Role and Performance

Who you report to affects how well your role as an ONN is developed and implemented. It also has a direct impact on how your performance will be measured and what the agreed-upon goals and objectives of your navigation responsibilities will be. No single specific designated person within a cancer center or cancer program serves as the supervisor of an ONN. The range unfortunately is broad. You might be reporting to a clinic manager, surgeon, medical oncologist, social worker, senior ONN, director of finance, administrator, tumor registrar, or even someone else. You need to know what *navigation* means to your supervisor. Did this person write your job description? Did he or she print it from a website because someone else said that it was an accurate job description for an ONN? Is this person measuring your performance based on return on investment (ROI) through patient retention of second-opinion patients? Or on patient satisfaction survey results? Or how well patients are maintained on their treatment plan to ensure that they are receiving treatment following NCCN treatment guidelines? Perhaps you will be measured based on marketing goals, and the ONN's role is to increase the volume of cancer patients treated at this cancer facility. Is the measurement based on the feedback from the doctors with whom you will be working?

You can see why it is important to get a clear picture of what your supervisor is thinking and planning for you. This is also a great time for negotiating. Do your homework in advance and request to see an annual report from the cancer center's CEO (Chief Executive Officer) or CAO (Chief Administrative Officer). Does the specific team you will be working with produce an annual report too? A breast center, colon center, prostate cancer center, or other large-volume cancer treatment team likely does. Read it to see what its performance has been over the last 3 years, whether navigation was even referenced in the report and in what way, and what the goals are for the time period that you will be entering as their new ONN. This is a time to be assertive in your discussions and provide some input that will be helpful. Above all else, make sure that the way your performance will be measured is something you agree is achievable. For example, if a primary measurement is the number of second-opinion patients who come for a consultation about their recommended cancer treatment and your task is to persuade those patients to stay and transfer their care to your treatment team, can you accomplish that? You need to be able to offer patients something they cannot receive where they have already been and were initially planning to get their care. This service available at your facility must be considered value added by patients.

What might be the difference is *you*. Other facilities may not have an ONN for patient navigation and support. Explaining to patients what you will be doing for them and how vital your role is for keeping them on track and preserving their milestones and life goals will likely do the trick in retaining patients. However, if you are working with a doctor who believes that all second-opinion patients should always be sent back to their initial cancer center where they were diagnosed and were originally planning to get their treatment, then you will be perpetually ambushed and unable to retain patients because the doctor will say there is no reason for the patient to stay at your facility. Another situation may be that the competitor facility hires a crackerjack ONN, and you lose your marketing edge if you are not the only ONN in town. You may be told that you are to bring in more residents from underserved neighborhoods for cancer screenings. Your ability to do this, however, will be based on the reasons why they aren't coming until now. If the barrier is transportation, myths, and/or misinformation, then you will likely have to find remedies for each. If you are not of the same race and ethnicity of the underserved population you are charged with recruiting, then again you may be set up to fail. You may need to recruit volunteers from that community to work with you and train them in order to gain trust within the community. You can see how important it is to know how you will be measured and how you can ensure that the goals you are given are really achievable by you.

Be careful what you take credit for too. Let's say that your cancer center hires a nationally renowned breast surgical oncologist. Women are coming to her supposedly for a second opinion, when really they are hoping to become her breast cancer patient. Then you cannot and should not be crediting yourself with retaining second-opinion patients when it actually was the new surgeon who became the (marketing) reason behind the new patients. You need to ensure that you are giving yourself credit for work that is yours.

Your supervisor may be familiar with the metrics that have been developed and implemented by AONN+ and plans to use some of those metrics to measure your performance. Chapter 5 will provide detailed information about these metrics. Review them and see if you want any to be used for measuring your performance.

Next, you need to know if your supervisor will go to bat for his employees or let them sink or swim on their own. You can learn this by interviewing others. When you are interviewed by a team, ask all team members their thoughts on what they believe is the most important function an ONN can fulfill on behalf of patients and on behalf of the multidisciplinary team. Write down all these answers to see who gets it and who doesn't. This type of information then needs to be discussed with your (potential) future supervisor. Ironing out these details in advance will make it easier for you to be successful.

If you have already been hired for the position and are experiencing challenges such as working with people who "don't get it," all is not lost. Meet now with team members and ask questions, record the responses, and meet with your supervisor to discuss this issue in more detail. You want everyone on the same page regarding what roles and responsibilities you do and don't have in the cancer center.

▶ Oncopolitics and Silo Structures within Your Organization[12]

Your role is unique in that you are likely involved with navigating and supporting patients across the continuum of care. But those you work with may not understand this. Surgeons do surgery. Medical oncologists select and administer chemotherapy and immunotherapy. Radiation oncologists give radiation therapy. Advance practice nurses serve as mid-level providers, addressing acute clinical situations such a fever spikes, wound care, and chemo side effects. Social workers can get patients on Medicaid coverage if they have no health insurance. The patient lay navigator is scheduling the patient for tests, consultations, and other appointments. Each of these individuals, who are just part of the overall team, are likely working in different departments, funded from different budgets. No single person oversees the entire team from a financial performance perspective. Although many cancer centers are working hard to break down these silos, it is difficult because they were established decades ago based on who holds the purse strings. And people don't like to part with money. It is that simple. Although you work together as a "team," your reporting structures are likely different and the source of your salary is very different. If someone just got laid off because of budget cuts in breast medical oncology and you just got hired in breast surgical oncology, eyebrows might be raised because people want to know if your new role will include navigating patients as they enter the next phase of treatment, that being chemotherapy in medical oncology.

Learn about the financial structure, organizational structure, and about the silos and oncopolitics that exist where you work. Don't plan or assume structures will change. Such changes take many years, sometimes decades. So before accepting any job, you need to feel comfortable that this is a structure you are willing to accept and then work within its constraints.

▶ Models of Patient Navigation[13]

When developing a patient navigation program within your cancer center, it is important to look at the organizational structure and determine what model will work best to address your patients' needs efficiently and effectively. The two current groupings for linking the navigator with the patient are:

- Matching navigator by tumor site (i.e., breast cancer)—a more clinically oriented approach
- Matching navigator by designated point of entry into the system—a more logistically driven method

There are variations within each grouping. In 2008, the Oncology Round Table, based on surveys and interviews of breast centers that are part of their membership, outlined various methods used within these models. The six models discussed in this section provide an overview of the most common variations within these two approaches. Dedicating patient navigators to a high-volume, low-acuity tumor site, such as breast cancer, remains the most common approach because this allows for higher patient loads per navigator. Some designate a navigator to focus on high-acuity complex patients who have the greatest need for services, such as those patients diagnosed with pancreatic cancer or head and neck cancer. Underserved cancer patients may also fall into such a category because of issues associated with noncompliance, literacy, lack of healthcare coverage, and other financial and culturally sensitive needs.

Over time the traditional navigation model has evolved to include a broad range of roles, all aimed at expanding access to care and improving the patient experience. Many navigators today are responsible for organizing and coordinating the multidisciplinary case conferences (which are sometimes referred to as tumor board meetings) and multiple clinics in the center. To increase the number of underserved women coming to the cancer center for screening tests and potentially diagnostic needs and cancer treatment, time is also dedicated to performing various outreach efforts in local communities by raising awareness and creating a process to make it easier to bring patients in for their routine cancer screening and clinical examination.

TABLES 3.1 and 3.2 present in chart format the two models referenced above.

The six models listed below provide an overview of the most common variations within the two approaches listed previously (matching navigator by tumor site and matching navigator by designated point of entry into the system):

- Model I: High-volume, low-acuity tumor sites—This is most commonly used for new navigation programs just getting started. Maintaining a high and consistently stable volume helps too in justifying the presence of a full-time navigator. Usually the nurse navigator begins intervention at the diagnostic evaluation process or at the time the breast biopsy in breast imaging is confirmed to be breast cancer.
- Model II: Low-volume, high-acuity tumor sites—This model is more commonly used in a clinical environment where the patients will need a great deal of time and resources to coordinate their care. Pancreatic cancer, lung cancer, head and neck cancer, and gynecologic oncology cancer patients are examples of these patient populations. Much of the care is provided in an inpatient hospital setting. Although volumes of patients are lower, they are known for being resource-intensive.
- Model III: All tumor sites—The cancer center determines that all patients are likely to benefit from patient navigation services to some degree. Individual navigator roles and responsibilities may actually vary based on the type of cancer that patients have. This can be a more complicated model if the navigators report to one leader overseeing patient navigation versus a clinician leader within the specific tumor site.
- Model IV: Multidisciplinary patient navigator—Such an individual is responsible for providing logistical support to multidisciplinary conferences and clinics to ensure that all the patient materials needed for case presentation are available and prepared for presentation, and the patient is informed of

TABLE 3-1 Group I: Navigators Designated by Tumor Site			
	Model I: High-Volume, Low-Acuity Tumor Sites	**Model II: Low-Volume, High-Acuity Tumor Sites**	**Model III: All Tumor Sites**
Description	Navigator assigned to high-volume, low-acuity tumor sites	Navigator assigned to low-volume, high-acuity tumor site(s)	Navigator assigned to provide coverage for all tumor sites
Rationale	Most commonly selected model because high-patient volumes tend to warrant assignment of a full-time equivalent	Patients with high levels of acuity tend to have a greater need for navigation services	Provides access to all cancer patients Recognizes universal need, benefit across tumor sites
Site	Breast cancer	Head and neck cancers GI cancers	All cancer types
Caveat	Although acuity is low, ensure that volumes are appropriate given navigator staffing	Level of frequency, intensity of navigation services likely to be high; consider role modifications	Varying patient volumes across groups may necessitate assigning several tumor sites per navigator

Data from Oncology Roundtable. Elevating the Patient Experience: Building Successful Patient Navigation, Multidisciplinary Care, and Survivorship Programs. Washington, DC: The Advisory Board Company; 2008.

the outcome of the team's discussion. The navigator assumes responsibility for time management of the conference itself and is also responsible for coordinating follow-up care for the patient based on the decisions and recommendations made by the team.

■ Model V: Patient navigators provide coverage via assigned physicians—This enables navigators to intervene when physicians identify specific patient needs. This model aims at increasing physicians' efficient use of time by intervening at the actual moment when needed, in addition to having the navigator perform the standard navigation role of identifying and eliminating barriers to care. To work well, standardization of this role is needed due to variation in the use of the navigator by various doctors.

■ Model VI: Patient navigator to address regional disparities—This really is where navigation was born (see the history of navigation section in Chapter 2). The navigator may be working in several different sites within a geographic region

TABLE 3-2 Group II: Navigators Designated by Patient Entry Point

	Model IV: Multidisciplinary Clinic	Model V: Physician Based	Model VI: Community Based
Description	Navigator assigned to tumor site-specific conference/clinic	Navigator assigned to work with several physicians	Navigator assigned to subset of population experiencing disparities in care
Rationale	Ensures timely case presentations, follow-up coordination	Provides assistance when need identified; opportunity to increase physician efficiency	Identifies and addresses gaps in access to and use of cancer service(s)
Site	Patient identified by referral, clinic visit	Patient identified by lead oncology physician	Patient identified in community by navigator
Caveat	Navigator clinic preparation, follow-up workload likely to vary by tumor site	Physician may request services beyond scope of navigator role Difficult to manage workload given physician variance	Funding commonly an issue; consider grant and foundation funding opportunities

Data from Oncology Roundtable. Elevating the Patient Experience: Building Successful Patient Navigation, Multidisciplinary Care, and Survivorship Programs. Washington, DC: The Advisory Board Company; 2008.

where patients are known to have significant gaps and barriers in accessing cancer services and care. This arrangement requires partnerships with other organizations. It also requires the navigator to develop site-specific programs focusing on promoting awareness, prevention, and screening. This navigator may transfer a patient to another navigator at the breast center once the patient has been diagnosed with breast cancer.

Whatever model your cancer center chooses to adopt, be sensitive to the fact that this takes time to create. Selecting a model is just one of the steps you will take when considering how to develop and implement a navigation program that works to address your patients' needs and supports the mission and scope of practice at your breast center. Plan carefully. It can be easy for a navigator to become overwhelmed because of high volume and failure to have resources in place to address the barriers as you identify them and work to eliminate them. Working efficiently is key. It will not always be possible to meet with patients face-to-face to carry out a certain task on their behalf. You may be communicating with them via phone or email.

You may even decide during the development process to implement two different models and compare the results in order to determine what model will serve your patients and organization best. Such work takes time; however, the final outcome should be a smooth delivery of care for your patients. Look at the current process, identify your barriers, select solutions (resources) to eliminate the barriers, measure how well the solutions are working, and revisit the process again. Your patients will be the benefactors of your hard work behind the scenes. As you adjust the process, you will find more time to work on additional ways to make their patient experience the best it can be.

Although this text is geared toward nurse navigators, some breast centers have opted to have other professionals, as well as lay persons, fulfilling some level of navigation for their patients. Who is doing the navigation and their educational background and skills have a direct impact on what level of navigation they can perform. The following sections examine six different categories of navigator role based on the individual's training and education.

Volunteer Navigator

During hard economic times, more and more institutions are revisiting the roles that volunteers fill and expanding those responsibilities to include direct patient contact. A volunteer can connect patients to educational information resources and community resources. Of course, there is no direct financial cost to the breast center, except for minimal human resources (HR) requirements such as tuberculosis (TB) testing, policy and procedure training for hazardous waste, and other universal training requirements of personnel who have physical contact with patients. Someone to supervise the volunteer is also required, as well as training this individual in carrying out the required tasks. Liability must be covered by the cancer center too in the event the volunteer navigator says or does something inappropriate (e.g., encourages a patient to see her surgeon instead of staying with the surgeon she has already seen and is planning to have surgery with). Determining how to measure a volunteer's effectiveness in doing these tasks must also be developed. You may have a volunteer(s) working with you to assist with clerical functions that otherwise you would be doing yourself (not a wise use of nursing resources). Volunteers, however, don't have to show up for work. Turnover can be a problem in some environments. It's harder to discipline someone who isn't doing a good job but wants to volunteer personal time.

Patient (Lay) Navigator

A patient (lay) navigator can connect patients with information and resources they need, and some institutions have decided to have only patient navigators. The costs usually are much less than those associated with a clinical professional. This individual can assist you in your work too and function as part of a team. The downside is that such navigators lack medical knowledge beyond their own experience (as many are cancer survivors themselves). Their value is certainly to be recognized because they can perform many navigation functions, particularly following up to make sure patients have kept their appointments and remained on track across the continuum of care. They can also connect patients to community resources and provide written educational materials and psychological support. Never underestimate their value.

Social Worker

Social workers' backgrounds allow them to assess patients for barriers and address their psychosocial needs as well as provide initial counseling. This level of healthcare professional may be less expensive than a registered nurse (RN) or advanced practice nurse (APN) but still have some level of clinical knowledge. They are usually very familiar with community resources and know how to use them. They are restricted in their level of medical knowledge and their ability to address treatment and symptom concerns that patients may have. Their expertise in getting patients qualified for some form of insurance coverage, such as Medical Assistance, and addressing the patients and families' psychosocial needs is superb. Today, however, there are fewer social workers available within hospitals and even within cancer centers. Their roles and responsibilities for some time have been difficult to articulate and when that happens, financial gurus can make poor decisions that such positions are no longer needed. Again, social workers, if you are fortunate enough to work with one on the team, can work with you so that the needs of your cancer patients are shared between you.

Oncology Nurse Navigator

This is the most common model today. The background of an RN, which an ONN has, provides patients with medically knowledgeable resources, and ONNs are trained to conduct a nursing assessment. As an ONN, you can play a larger role in patients' care because you have a license and have taken care of cancer patients prior to becoming an ONN. You are familiar with the diagnosis and treatment planning process. You can also refer patients to support services as needed. Although you may lack familiarity with community resources initially, you can learn this information relatively quickly by interacting with the oncology social worker on the team as well as visiting these resources in the community yourself. You can also place phone calls to national advocacy organizations to introduce yourself and learn what resources they have to support your patient population. This model is a more costly model than one that includes nonclinical individuals, but it remains the most popular one adopted by cancer centers today. More than 80% of navigators currently working for cancer centers are RNs functioning as ONNs.

Advanced Practice Nurse

APNs' backgrounds tend to bring more credibility to the navigator role from a physician's perspective. There is also the potential to be able to bill for navigator services within the nursing model of care. APNs can play a larger role, even beyond that of the RN if needed. Once they have has learned what support services are available within the institution and local community, they can refer patients. This model is the most expensive, and it can be difficult to justify the higher cost above an RN level unless the cancer center implements a way to bill for APN services. Of navigators currently working in cancer centers, about 10% are APNs. Nurse practitioners are usually doing dual roles of seeing patients as a mid-level provider while also fulfilling some specific navigation roles for patients and their families.

Navigators by Another Name

Not all people who are navigators are called navigators, which can make it complicated for team members to understand the role of navigators. It can also be confusing for patients. Sometimes an ONN is referred to as a care coordinator, clinical triage nurse (working in the scheduling office to review pathology, scans, and other tests and determine what the correct next steps are for getting patients diagnosed and/or efficiently treated), or multidisciplinary team coordinator, in addition to other names.

Someone may be called a navigator but frankly not perform navigation functions. This can happen for several reasons. The first is that someone read the CoC standards and realized that a navigation program is a required standard to achieve in order to become accredited by the CoC. However, the standard explicitly states that a *navigation program* must be in place; it doesn't recommend hiring a navigator and then considering your institution as having a navigator program. Some people, including those in leadership positions, are confused about the differences between a navigator and a navigation program.

Another reason is lack of buy-in. Your job description may say that you are a nurse navigator, and it may be accurate for your role performing as an ONN. But no one among the team members, your supervisor, and others know exactly what your tasks should be. The job description was solely used to get the job posted and you hired. Again, don't let that happen to you. You want to fulfill the roles and responsibilities of an ONN and not complete the tasks no one else wants to do. Always be sure you are working to the highest level of your licensure.

▶ How the Oncology Care Setting Influences the Structure and Processes of Navigation

No two navigation programs are exactly alike. Some may share similar structures or principles, but if you look for a navigation program, find one at another cancer center, and think it will fit perfectly into your institution, think again. There are many reasons why the transfer will be difficult at best: the differences in overall organizational structure and oncopolitics, and continued confusion about the goals of navigation. Be patient and don't give up. Remember, you are the patient's advocate. Your patients need you.

Different cancer care settings influence the structure and process of navigation. You might be working in an urban teaching hospital, a rural community hospital, or perhaps an oncology care model (OCM) within a physician practice. Each one has its own structure. Each one is very different from the others. Urban teaching facilities commonly see a relatively large volume of underserved patients who live within walking distance of the institution. These patients usually have several other unaddressed comorbidities, rarely if ever seek medical care, have financial concerns that are significant, and may be culturally biased against seeking medical care for fear of being "experimented on." Such cancer centers also draw patients who have more complex cancers. For example, a 46-year-old woman with a stage 2 breast cancer can usually be treated in a community setting. If this same patient is pregnant with her first child, you now have two patients who are best cared for in a teaching facility or academic facility and not a community setting, where there is a lack of expertise for this type of situation. The volume of specific types of cancers, such as breast, colorectal, thoracic, and prostate, will likely be large enough to have ONNs dedicated to cancer specific multidisciplinary teams. Keep all this in mind when you are interviewing for an open position in this type of setting.

Urban teaching facilities commonly are heavily involved in offering clinical trials to patients. They have a large number of residents and medical students who are learning and also become part of the oncology multidisciplinary team. They are only involved for a relatively short period of time before they are rotated to the next element of their learning in medical school there. You will be working with them, and this is a golden opportunity for *you* to teach medical students and residents about oncology navigation. Remember, they will one day graduate and be out in the workforce themselves as doctors. Take advantage of teaching them about this important element of the cancer care continuum so that they under-stand it, value it, and want to incorporate it into their eventual model of care. Keep in mind too that these types of facilities usually have a lot of special services within their own doors—nutrition; cancer rehabilitation; psychologists/therapists; housing for families while their loved one is treated; genetics counseling; palliative care; hospice care; interventional radiology; organ-specific tumor board meetings; all aspects of treatment, including surgical oncology, medical oncology, radiation oncology, and so on. You will likely have a role in screening patients for clinical trials perhaps too.

Now let's talk about community hospitals. Seventy percent of cancer treat-ments are provided currently at community hospitals. These facilities can be within a city/town or can be in a very rural setting. Urban/suburban community hospitals usually don't have residency training programs. They also don't usually see and treat complex cancer patients (like someone diagnosed with pancreatic cancer needing a Whipple procedure). Most of their patients are early diagnosed cancer patients who are relatively straightforward to treat. They may or may not have fewer barriers to care. Their volumes of cancer patients will be less than large urban teaching hospitals or academic cancer centers. You, as an ONN, may be seeing ev-eryone diagnosed with cancer because there isn't adequate volume of one specific type of cancer to warrant hiring tumor-specific ONNs. This setting can be quite challenging because it requires you to stay up to date on treatment modalities, the newest cutting-edge research that has been published, what clinical trials might be offered in this setting, and so on. The volume will be higher when simply looking at numbers of patients you are supporting, but likely with a lower acuity than at an urban teaching facility.

If the community cancer center is in a very rural setting, however, there are even more things that need to be considered when navigating patients who, from the beginning, have geographic barriers. This facility might be the only one for 200 miles, which means patients travel a long distance for everything. They may not be able to take time off from work as often as needed to get the preferred standard of care. Some patients may sign up for mastectomy surgery when they need only a lumpectomy for a very small tumor because they cannot take off a lot of time to get radiation after their breast-conserving surgery. These patients usually have limited resources, do not seek medical care regularly, and may also be diagnosed with a more advanced cancer than hoped. This is where you will want to spend time in the community where these patients live and work to learn about their daily challenges, see about developing advocacy organizations to help support their needs (such as a place for the patient and family to stay when the patient has surgery and the family cannot afford to go to a hotel for several days). This will be the first of what hopefully will become the formation of many partnerships to support this rural community, accomplished with your help. You will want to exert the same effort if you are planning to work in an urban setting.

Hopefully you will have someone within the facility where you will be working to fill you in on what types of community resources are available as well as what resources are still lacking. Don't assume because there isn't a solution to a barrier, like lack of transportation, that there never will be. You need to take it upon yourself to see if you can find that solution, whatever it may be, through advocacy efforts as well as grant applications.

Community facilities, whether located in an urban, suburban, or rural area, usually need to make referrals for specialty services such as genetics counseling, nutrition, cancer rehabilitation, and so on. You will have an instrumental role in making sure that the services patients need are obtained through some referral mechanism and provided in a timely manner. This means getting to know these specialty service professionals so you can pick up the phone, call them by their first name, ask them how they weekend was, and request an urgent referral for genetics counseling and testing of newly diagnosed breast cancer patients because the type of surgery they will be scheduled for depends directly on whether they carry a breast cancer gene mutation.

Now let's talk about the OCM. The OCM is about delivering, ensuring, and measuring quality cancer care. In short, it is a patient-focused system of delivering quality cancer care that is coordinated and efficient. It is designed to meet the needs of patients, payers, and providers.

You may work in this type of practice model and perform navigation responsibilities that you have been learning about. Keeping patients on track for their care, making sure they don't drop through the cracks, as well as looking at their short- and long-term navigation needs will be important tasks for you. You might even have some underserved patients who become part of the case mix of this practice because of negotiations that the practice leaders have made with Medicaid or other health insurers. These patients will likely be followed longer after their treatment is completed and relationships with primary care providers becomes part of the structure.

OCMs were developed by the Medicare and Medicaid Innovation Program, and they are likely the future of oncology care. Some of the key aspects of the OCM mean that a patient's cancer care will be:

- Coordinated with the central focus on patients and their entire medical condition.
- Optimized based on evidence-based medicine to produce quality outcomes.
- Accessible and efficient, with treatment provided in the highest quality, lowest cost setting for the patient.
- Delivered in a patient-centric, caring environment that optimizes patient satisfaction.
- Improved continuously by measuring and benchmarking results against other facilities providing care so that best practices raise the bar in delivering care.

I hope you can see that navigation is a key element of accomplishing the above model of care. You, as an ONN, are integral to the team and to the patients.

▶ How Many Navigators Are Needed to Navigate the Patients at My Cancer Facility?

If I had a dollar for every time I have been asked this question I would be very rich. Many factors go into calculating how many navigators a cancer center or organ-specific cancer program needs to navigate its patients effectively and efficiently across all phases of care. The answer depends on the type of cancer, its stages, volume of underserved patients, barriers that have an impact on patients' treatment, financial toxicities they will likely incur without your help, patients' severity of illness, patients' complexity of care, what comorbidities patients have prior to their cancer diagnosis, and what level of family support they have.

To determine the answer to this question requires having accurate data, and keep in mind that this data will likely change over time. For example, perhaps your institution receives a grant to promote lung nodule screening, and your cancer center just hired a new thoracic surgical oncologist so that your facility can begin diagnosing and treating individuals with lung cancer. Your center wasn't able to offer these services, except chemotherapy, previously. This means that you need to see and hopefully even be part of writing the business plan and the grant that reflects, from the community needs assessment, how many consumers are likely to be screened, and how many are likely to be diagnosed earlier than they are presently, thus enabling them to have surgery for their lung cancer. This impacts your case mix significantly if things go as hoped and planned. You or one of your fellow ONNs will be adding to their acuity mix and, if volumes are high enough, becoming a dedicated ONN for lung cancer patients. Don't assume that once the right number of ONNs is calculated and implemented that leadership, as well as you and your navigation colleagues, maintain the current volume for the coming years. How efficiently you are functioning as an ONN is a critical measurement in this situation too. Are you doing re-work? Are you creating a workday schedule that is the most efficient that can be created to get your work done?

I have learned, over my more than 45 years in the medical field, that if I give someone 5 tasks to do and he or she has 8 hours to do them, he or she will more than likely use the entire 8 hours, or close to it, to complete this work. If I give the same individual 10 tasks to do, he or she would have probably accomplished and completed this work too in those same 8 hours. Efficiency can be influenced by the amount of time someone is given to perform tasks. When it comes to navigating cancer patients, however, it isn't like putting a widget on an object as it goes along a conveyor belt or like candy being covered in chocolate. (Remember the famous episode from the *I Love Lucy* show, when Lucy and Ethel worked a candy line?) Such work is very predictable and easy to measure (except for Lucy and Ethel, that is). You know the speed of the conveyor belt, how many widgets you have to place, and how much time you have to do it. Of course, people aren't widgets and you are not standing in front of a conveyor belt. Each patient is unique and has a unique disease acuity, which can and often does change as he or she progresses through various phases of treatment. This is why cancer patient acuity needs to be studied and calibrated thoughtfully. AONN+ recognizes that it is not easy to do. Many hospital administers, think, however, that getting the right number of navigators based solely on the number of cancer patients being treated should be simple. Well, it isn't. You may be working at the same pace you have for a long time, only to learn that perhaps you have filled your day with only the 5 tasks mentioned above. Now you are told that, based on newly calculated acuity scores, you will have your work doubled. Don't assume that you can't get it done or that you are being treated unfairly. First, see how the calculation was made, then take a serious, thoughtful, and objective look at where you can regain efficiency within your day or week.

Look too at how clerical tasks are performed. If you are standing at a fax machine for 30 minutes a day, this is time wasted unless you are able to multi-task and make patient calls, review pathology results, or do someone else that needs to be done by an ONN at that same time. Always bring to the attention of your supervisor the amount of time spent doing clerical tasks. Even calculate how much money it is costing the institution for you to do these clerical duties. For example, let's say that you spend 30 minutes a day, 5 days a week standing at the fax machine without the ability to multi-task during that time. If you get 4 weeks' vacation, you work 48 weeks annually. This means that you are spending 120 hours a year standing at the fax machine. If your salary is $30 an hour and your benefits are 34% of your salary, your benefits equal $10.20 per hour. When you add the salary and benefits, you have an hourly rate of $40.20. Multiply this by 120 and you have $4,820. This is how much the institution is spending on you to stand at a fax machine. A volunteer doing the faxing means that you can perform the tasks that are in keeping with your medical background and licensure.

Now you may also be in a situation where the acuity score shows you are exceeding your expected capacity of work. Does that mean you give up some portion of your patients to be navigated by someone else on the team? The answer depends on many factors. Again, look at how your time has been spent and determine if you feel heavily burdened. Some people love being busy every single minute of their day. I am one of those people. Others do not, and that needs to be respected with lunch breaks and a 15-minute break both in the morning and in the afternoon. That usually equals a whole hour of time to get recharged and refreshed.

Because you are reading this book, you are likely new to the world of oncology navigation, and when you begin your ONN role, you may be slower than you eventually will be once you are proficient in performing certain tasks and functions. Be sure to work with your supervisor so that your workload grows over an agreed-upon designated length of time rather than expecting you to hit the ground running and doing everything perfectly and proficiently. I would be remiss if I didn't mention that not all people are proficient professionals. It simply isn't their strength. I have worked with such individuals in various settings over my career, and although I feel very frustrated with what I consider to be a slow performer or someone less efficient than desirable, he or she they may not be able to change. Taking a course on maximizing efficiency and effectiveness helps some people. Learning tricks of the trade from experienced ONNs certainly can be beneficial too. You might be really talented at specific aspects of navigation and less proficient at other components. You may be able to work with your navigation team and create a special workflow process that maximizes your strengths and that of others, while having those tasks that you do not handle as well become the work of someone who loves that part of the job. You need to be mindful that you do not dump work that you don't do well (and probably don't enjoy as much) on a coworker. It will come back to bite you in the end. Enough said on that subject.

▶ AONN+ Navigation Acuity Measures

You will be pleased to know that AONN+ has taken the necessary steps on your behalf to create a task force that is dedicated to measuring acuity. The ability to calculate the level of care needed for a particular patient across the care continuum could prove invaluable for oncology navigation programs. Through a collaboration with *astellas*, AONN+ is working to develop, standardize, and implement an evidence-based oncology navigation acuity tool that is intended to be applicable across all settings and types of navigation. This work officially began in 2018, although it was discussed by the AONN+ Leadership Council for some time prior to this date. It will take some time to master its use, but we are well underway to achieving the goals that are needed to answer the question posed earlier—how many ONNs do I need to navigate my cancer patients at my cancer facility? Remember, this number must be somewhat fluid because case mix of the patient population changes over time, decisions made by leadership regarding what types of cancer patients they want to treatment also changes, which brings in the marketing department and the hiring of medical staff and others to manage this new patient population. There may even be situations in which decisions are made to discontinue the care and treatment of certain types of cancer patients. Such decisions are commonly based on financial outcomes and not clinical outcomes. The acuity tool is aimed at evaluating each patient's level of need based on the intensity and severity of the disease and, by doing so, gaining the ability to assess a navigator's caseload more accurately. In short, the proposed tool "will characterize the intensity of the navigation workload, aid in the allocation of navigation resources, and measure the effectiveness of navigation on patient outcomes." However, *acuity*, as the team defined it, "is not productivity." It is an attempt to balance the navigator's workload while also demonstrating the value of navigation in a quantitative fashion and fulfilling the navigator's role of removing barriers to care.[14]

The proposed acuity measurement will incorporate navigation core competencies, national oncology standards, and the AONN+ standardized navigation metrics to provide a validated resource that fosters sustainability in navigation programs. Applicable across settings and roles, the tool will be uncomplicated and easy to implement for navigation teams, bringing them closer to the goal of providing safe, effective, and efficient care.[14]

Visit the AONN+ website (www.aonnonline.org) to learn more about the Navigation Acuity Toolkitand watch for email updates as well as presentations by the task force dedicated to this work. The task force provides to AONN+ members information in the form of webinars and/or a presentation at an AONN+ conference. This is exciting work!

▶ Summary

This chapter dug deeper into your future roles and responsibilities as an ONN. I also talked about the various models of navigation and focused on navigation settings and types and volumes of cancer patients. I discussed the importance of finding your place successfully within a multidisciplinary team as well as the importance of knowing and understanding who your supervisor is and how that individual will measure your performance. You will be working with other professionals who may have specific roles within the navigation space, and these responsibilities, tasks, and functions need to be understood and spelled out, and preferably documented.

Learning boundaries is key to your success as well. Clear delineation of your responsibilities versus others on the team need to be explicitly stated and agreed upon, hopefully before you launch into your new role as an ONN. I provided an example of how this might be accomplished. It is impossible to escape oncopolitics, and I hope I provided you an inside look at what that means and how to navigate around what could be land mines in your way to becoming the best ONN you can possibly be for your patients.

You have a vital role in navigating patients along their cancer journey as efficiently as possible. You too must work efficiently to accomplish your work and meet expectations. If additional tasks are given to you, take the time to perform operations management to revise how you currently get your work done, and do this before someone else decides to look more closely at how you spend your time. It is less stressful to do a self-evaluation than to have someone hovering over you watching what you do.

Finally, I examined the question that I am asked most often—how many navigators do I need to navigate the patients in my cancer facility? Continue to learn more about the progress being made on your behalf regarding the development and eventual availability for implementation of an acuity system that will answer that critical question.

Let's take a look at operations management next in Chapter 4.

References

1. AONN+ website. https://aonnonline.org/education/learning-guides/22-learning-guide -professional-roles-and-responsibilities. Accessed May 8, 2019.
2. Willis A, Reed E, Pratt-Chapman M, et al. Development of a framework for patient navigation: Delineating roles across navigator types. *J Oncol Navig Surviv.* 2013;4:20–26.
3. Brown CG, Cantril C, McMullen L, et al. Oncology nurse navigator role delineation study: An Oncology Nursing Society report. *Clin J Oncol Nurs.* 2012;16:581–585.
4. Seek A, Hogle W. Modeling a better way: Navigating the healthcare system for patients with lung cancer. *Clin J Oncol Nurs.* 2007;11:81–85.
5. Blaseg K. Getting started as a nurse navigator. In: Blaseg K, Daugherty P, Gamblin K, eds. *Oncology Nurse Navigation Delivering Patient-Centered Care Across the Continuum.* Pittsburgh, PA: Oncology Nursing Society, 2014:20–42.
6. Vargas RB, Ryan GW, Jackson CA, et al. Characteristics of the original patient navigation programs to reduce disparities in the diagnosis and treatment of breast cancer. *Cancer.* 2008;113:426–433.
7. Fillion L, Cook S, Veillette A, et al. Professional navigation framework: Elaboration and validation in a Canadian context. *Oncol Nurs Forum.* 2012;39:E58–E69.
8. Doll R, Barroetavena MC, Ellwood AL, et al. The cancer care navigator: Toward a conceptual framework for a new role in oncology. *Oncol Exchange.* 2007;6(4):28–33.
9. Christensen D, Bellomo C. Using a nurse navigation pathway in the timely care of oncology patients. *J Oncol Navig Surviv.* 2014;5(3):13–18.
10. Shockney L. Understand cancer survivorship. Presented at Wellspan Oncology Conference, York, PA, October 19, 2018.
11. National Comprehensive Cancer Network. www.nccn.org. Accessed May 5, 2019
12. Shockney L. Navigating oncopolitics. Presented at the Spring 2018 AONN+ Conference. Power-Point presentation available for members on the AONN+ website. www.aonnonline.org. Accessed May 27, 2019.
13. Shockney L. *Becoming a Breast Cancer Nurse Navigator.* City, ST: Jones & Bartlett Publishing, 2011. https://aonnonline.org/expert-commentary/navigation-and-survivorship-news/596-insights -into-navigation-too-many-patients-and-not-enough-time. Accessed June 3, 2019.

© mevoo/Shutterstock

CHAPTER 4

A Prerequisite to Navigating Your Oncology Patient Effectively and Efficiently

▶ Experience Your Cancer Facility through the Eyes of a Patient[1]

I know you are anxious to get started in your new role as an oncology nurse navigator (ONN). Before you can become an ONN proficient in your work, however, you need to experience your cancer center, and in particular the clinic or specialty cancer program (such as a breast center or colon cancer center) from the other side—as a patient, not literally but figuratively. Travel the same journey your patient takes. Walk in the patient's shoes. Don't assume you know all the steps even if you've previously been working in your cancer center and with the same team you have worked with for several years. Even I was surprised when I did this process myself. What I thought was working okay wasn't working all the time. What I assumed was done by others wasn't what I thought at all. You will have a bird's eye view if you spend some time observing the process yourself and documenting what you see. Before long, the barriers to inefficiency and the communication gaps will stare you in the face. *Do not intervene* while doing this observation either, although it will be tempting. Record it just as it is presently.

If your role begins at the time the patient is diagnosed, begin at the point the patient is called back after having had a screening test that warrants more diagnostic workup. Create a flowchart and look at each step. Put a time line to what you see. Remember to record the "who does what, when, where, how, and why." Be prepared to be surprised. This process is known as operations management. The Wikipedia definition of operations management is: "... an area of management concerned with designing and controlling the process of production and redesigning business operations in the production of goods or services. It involves the responsibility of ensuring that business operations are efficient in terms of using as few resources as needed and effective in terms of meeting customer requirements. Operations management is primarily concerned with planning, organizing and supervising in the contexts of production, manufacturing or the provision of services." Now you might think that this couldn't apply to an environment where patients are receiving care. However, health care is the business of providing patient care. Unfortunately, it is also where people in charge of structures and processes are medically trained and don't have business education and/or training. Although it certainly is true that we need to look at each patient as unique, the processes whereby we provide care should be as streamlined as possible.

In your operations management process, you want to identify where there are delays, duplications of effort, and risk of something falling through the cracks and not being done at all. Identify processes that are outdated and inefficient, and look for electronic methods to replace them. As the new ONN, you should not be serving as a Band-Aid for a broken process.

▶ Documenting the Patient Flow Process

This chapter introduces various tools and resources to help you get started on your success or to further enhance your success as an ONN. As mentioned previously, it is very hard to navigate for someone else without knowing the patient care flow process yourself. A key component of your job focuses on ensuring that patients are diagnosed and treated in a timely manner. This means that you need to know how efficiently the current care delivery model in your breast center works and identify ways in which it can be improved.

TABLE 4-1 provides a template for recording information about your patient flow process. The comments section allows you to record information that may help you to identify barriers that are prolonging the time between one step and the next along the continuum of care. Maybe you note a time lag between the patient's postoperative appointment with the surgeon and her appointment to see a medical oncologist next about systemic treatment. Investigating who is responsible for making that medical oncology appointment and when it is arranged can give you key information about shortening that time. If medical oncology appointments aren't scheduled until after patients see their surgeon for their postoperative evaluation, then the time lag could be several weeks. If the medical oncology consultation was scheduled proactively at the time that the surgery was arranged, then the time lag can be dramatically shortened.

You may want to include additional steps in the process, such as notifying the clinical trials office of a potential patient for a research study, referring the patient to be fitted for a wig, signing her up to join a cancer support group, and having additional diagnostic studies performed. The chart in Table 4-1 is a starting point for you to create your own patient flowchart that matches the processes of care in your setting. I chose the breast center because this is the setting I work in. Keep Table 4-1 in mind as you read the examples on the following pages and learn how implementing a small change in the process can have a positive impact on patient care. Also, follow

TABLE 4-1 Flowchart Depicting the Current Patient Flow Process in a Breast Center

Process Being Performed	Average Number of Days to Next Step	Comments
Recruitment of patient for screening mammogram	_____	_____
Screening mammogram performed	_____	_____
Screening mammogram read by radiologist	_____	_____
Patient informed of abnormal results	_____	_____
Patient scheduled for diagnostic mammogram/ ultrasound	_____	_____
Referring physician notified	_____	_____
Patient scheduled for biopsy, educated regarding procedure	_____	_____
Biopsy performed in breast imaging setting	_____	_____
Biopsy results available from pathology	_____	_____
Referring physician informed that results show breast cancer	_____	_____
Patient informed that pathology results show cancer	_____	_____
Surgical consultation scheduled	_____	_____
Patient seen by a breast surgeon for consultation	_____	_____

(continues)

TABLE 4-1 Flowchart Depicting the Current Patient Flow Process in a Breast Center   *(continued)*

Process Being Performed	Average Number of Days to Next Step	Comments
Magnetic resonance imaging (MRI) requested and ordered (if needed)	_____	_____
Results of MRI known and reviewed by surgeon	_____	_____
Plastic surgery consultation arranged because of MRI findings	_____	_____
Breast cancer surgery scheduled	_____	_____
Preoperative teaching for patient scheduled	_____	_____
Preoperative tests and History & Physical scheduled	_____	_____
Surgery performed, e.g., mast with DIEP flap	_____	_____
Pathology available from surgery	_____	_____
Receptors from pathology available from surgery	_____	_____
Other genomic tests ordered (if appropriate)	_____	_____
Patient returns for postopertive visit	_____	_____
Patient scheduled for medical oncology consultation (if needed)	_____	_____
Patient seen by medical oncologist (if appropriate)	_____	_____

Process Being Performed	Average Number of Days to Next Step	Comments
Patient has staging workup (if needed)	_____	_____
Results of staging workup available and reviewed by oncologist	_____	_____
Patient receives teaching about chemotherapy regimen	_____	_____
Patient begins chemotherapy regimen	_____	_____
Cycle 1	_____	_____
Cycle 2	_____	_____
Cycle 3	_____	_____
Cycle 4	_____	_____
Patient scheduled for radiation oncology consultation (if needed)	_____	_____
Patient seen by radiation oncologist (if needed)	_____	_____
Education about radiation therapy conducted with patient	_____	_____
Simulation for radiation therapy scheduled	_____	_____
Simulation for radiation performed	_____	_____
Radiation therapy begins	_____	_____
Radiation therapy completed	_____	_____

(continues)

| | Average Number of | |
Process Being Performed	Days to Next Step	Comments
Patient scheduled to see medical oncologist for hormonal therapy	_____	_____
Patient begins hormonal therapy	_____	_____
Patient monitored for adherence to hormonal therapy	_____	_____
Patient scheduled for follow-up appointments and tests as needed	_____	_____

TABLE 4-1 Flowchart Depicting the Current Patient Flow Process in a Breast Center   *(continued)*

several patients, each with a different clinical scenario, from beginning to end. It will take time to record all this information, but you will be glad you did when you finish your operations management data collection process.

TABLE 4-2 presents specific phases of care, measured in time, for you to see how establishing a baseline of information, implementing a change, and remeasuring the process of care results in an improvement that can be documented and, best of all, implemented as the new standard of care delivery in your setting. Remember, you don't want to be functioning as a Band-Aid in this broken system.

By making changes when the medical oncology appointment is scheduled, as shown in Table 4-2, the patient can start chemotherapy 3 weeks sooner. Again, given my specialty is breast cancer, I am providing you examples that I have personally experienced.

Now that you've had an opportunity to give some thought to the patient flow process, let's examine the impact of making just a small change in the care delivery process on improving efficiency, effectiveness, and overall quality of care. Examine the scenario in **TABLE 4-3**. You can see that medical oncology appointments are taking 3 to 4 weeks before an appointment slot was available. See how the scheduling process was changed based on this type of operations management results so that patients were not delayed in getting their medical oncology appointments and thus were getting underway with their next phase of treatment.

By the way, the Band-Aid method would have resulted in you calling each medical oncologist and asking if any of them can accept an add-on patient to their schedule within the next few days. That would be time consuming and probably not very fruitful. In addition, you would have a very worried patient who would need

TABLE 4-2 Comparison of Time Lag by Making a Change in the Scheduling Process for Postoperative Medical Oncology Appointments

Old Process	New Process
The patient was seen by a breast surgeon on 5/30/2019, and at the end of the consultation the patient scheduled for surgery to be performed on 6/21/2019.	The patient was seen by a breast surgeon on 5/30/2019, and at the end of the consultation the patient was scheduled for surgery 6/21/2019. Patient also scheduled for medical oncology appointment for 6/30/2019.
Surgery performed 6/21/2019.	Surgery performed 6/21/2019.
Pathology results available 6/26/2019.	Pathology results available 6/26/2019.
Patient seen by surgeon for postoperative appointment 6/27/2019.	Patient seen by surgeon for postoperative appointment 6/27/2019.
Upon departure from postoperative appointment, the patient scheduled for medical oncology appointment 7/23/2019 (this was the first available appointment available).	No need to schedule medical oncology appointment upon leaving clinic because it was proactively scheduled when the surgery date was scheduled.
Medical oncology consultation performed 7/23/2019.	Medical oncology consultation performed 6/30/2019.
Chemotherapy begins 8/1/2019.	Chemotherapy begins 7/6/2019.

constant consoling, having heard that she needs chemotherapy first and is not even a surgical candidate at this time.

Examine the next opportunity for improving efficiency and expediting the patient's care and treatment in Table 4-3. The time difference for getting the patient underway for treatment is significant—3 weeks. From the perspective of the patient, it is vital to get treatment started as soon as possible. Inflammatory breast cancer is, from its onset, classified as stage 3 breast cancer. It is the one time that systemic treatment must start quickly. By recognizing at the time that the pathology results are available that the patient has inflammatory breast cancer, steps can be taken to fast-track her to medical oncology to start neoadjuvant chemotherapy. It can be quite distressing for a patient to see a surgeon first and be told that she is not operable, and that she needs systemic treatment before surgery can be considered. Her anxiety can increase still more if she has to wait several days a week before seeing a medical oncologist. In addition, her clinical outcome may be worse due to a long delay.

In this scenario, you are making sure the care is provided more efficiently and you are also addressing the patient's psychological needs. The patient can see the

TABLE 4-3 Utilizing Pathology Information from the Biopsy to Schedule Appointments Efficiently

Old Process	New Process
Biopsy results confirm inflammatory breast cancer 6/2/2019.	Biopsy results confirm inflammatory breast cancer 6/2/2019.
Patient scheduled for surgical consultation 6/10/2019. Upon consulting with the patient, the surgeon refers the patient to medical oncology due to the patient not being a surgical candidate at this time.	
Patient referred to medical oncology for consultation about neoadjuvant chemotherapy upon leaving the clinic on 6/10/2019.	Patient scheduled for urgent medical oncology consultation by scheduler based on the ONN's clinical triage of this case. An urgent medical oncology appointment slot is built into the scheduling system based on the frequency of needing to perform neoadjuvant chemotherapy before surgery. Two appointment slots a week were made available based on the operations management results.
Patient seen by medical oncologist 6/26/2019.	Patient seen by medical oncologist 6/5/2019.
Staging workup completed 6/30/2019.	Staging workup completed 6/9/2019. It included patient meeting the surgeon for clinical assessment before chemotherapy started.
Neoadjuvant chemotherapy begins 7/3/2019.	Neoadjuvant chemotherapy begins 6/12/2019.

breast surgeon during the staging workup phase or even during the first week of chemotherapy. The surgeon can examine her and continue to see her during her chemotherapy treatments with the goal of doing her mastectomy surgery when chemotherapy is completed and the dermal lymphatics of the skin of the breast have been cleared of cancer.

Building in urgent medical oncology appointment slots for patients who need neoadjuvant chemotherapy improves the patient's clinical outcome and psychological well-being. This was only possible because you performed an operations management process by creating a flowchart and identifying where delays in the process, risk of the patient dropping through the cracks, and other inefficiencies and solving them upfront by reworking the patient flow process.

▶ Software to Help You Track Your Patients and Produce Reports

As you navigate more and more of your patients across the continuum of care, it will not take very long for you to begin feeling overwhelmed with keeping track of test results and the next steps you need to take to facilitate assessments, care, and treatment. You might begin using a Kardex system to record information. (For those of you who have been oncology nurses for as long as I have, you probably just groaned!) This approach can quickly become cumbersome and at times frustrating, especially if you are responsible for a large number of patients. One solution is to capture the information electronically via computer and let the software remind you what needs to happen next on any given day for your patients. Using navigation software can also ease the process when you need to be away and someone else is filling in for you.

Most cancer centers today use electronic patient records, if they are not, they should be. Depending on the type of software system used, you can look to see if you can create a dedicated section of the software for recording your navigation information. It is ideal when the information you record is accessible to the rest of the team members taking care of the patients so that they too can see the milestones, life goals, and specific interventions you have done and will do for patients.

If your center does not use electronic patient records, consider using at least an Excel spreadsheet to record your information. We cannot manage what we do not measure. (Remember this quote from me.) An Excel program can help you produce summary reports, for example, the number of new patients you are navigating, the number of patients who had barriers and what the barriers were, what you did to resolve those barriers, the number of no-shows for specific appointments, and so on.

The next section is a case study that walks you through a patient's entire journey, from the point of abnormal mammogram through the completion of her breast cancer treatment.

▶ Navigation Example across the Continuum: A Case Study

This case study uses the letters B, E, T, S, and Q, a system I created a few years ago, to help define what the navigator should be identifying within any specific phase of a patient's care or treatment.[1] This technique may not be scientific, but I have found it helpful:

B   Barriers: Define the barriers to progressing the patient from one phase of care or treatment to another.

E   Education: Educate the patient.

T   Tracking: Track data to ensure quality control.

S   Scheduling: Schedule steps that must take place to navigate her to the next step.

Q   Quality: Identify ways to measure performance through the application of quality measurements.

Details are key here. As mentioned before, navigation cannot be done by one person. Knowing who is involved, what their responsibilities are, and how to communicate with them is critical to your success as an ONN.

While evaluating this process from an operations management perspective, pay attention to the following:

- Duplication of effort
- Delays in the delivery of care
- Whether the appropriate person is responsible for the appropriate task based on skill
- Knowledge, salary, and time allotted to accomplish it

Anticipate some changes in workflow as one of the outcomes of conducting this important analysis. The end result should be a well-oiled machine that functions smoothly, consistently, and reliably.

This case study serves as an example of what your role as navigator might be as you navigate a patient across the continuum:

Screening mammogram (bi-rad 4c) Diagnostic imaging Core biopsy

A 48-year-old patient came in for her routine screening mammogram on Thursday, April 2. She had no breast abnormalities to report. Her films were read the following day, and a spiculated mass, measuring 1.3 cm, was noted in the upper-outer quadrant of the left breast. The breast-imaging scheduler called the patient to inform her she needed additional imaging done. She was scheduled to return on Monday, April 6. The call was transferred to the navigator, who did the following:

- Explained what a bi-rad 4 c score on breast imaging means and what the likelihood is that the biopsy might show cancer (80% risk of being cancer)
- Inquired about medications the patient may be taking that might interfere with performing a biopsy the same day
- Educated the patient about diagnostic mammograms, breast ultrasound, spot films, and core biopsy procedure
- Reiterated time to arrive on Monday, and requested that the patient bring a family member or a friend to drive her home because a biopsy may be performed the same day
- Inquired if there were any barriers that would prevent the patient from keeping her appointment for Monday (child care, co-payments, fear, transportation, work requirements, etc.)

    S   Patient needs to be scheduled for diagnostic mammogram, possibly ultrasound and core/stereo biopsy (factor in questions about blood thinners, local anesthetic).

    B   Assess for barriers related to compliance with keeping appointment for diagnostic evaluation (getting off work, child care, co-payments, understanding the importance of keeping this appointment).

    E   Educate patient about meaning of bi-rad score of 4 c; the purpose of additional imaging studies, such as spot films and ultrasound; the biopsy procedure; and how biopsy results will be provided to her.

T   Record the date of screening mammogram and date for diagnostic evaluation and biopsy.

Q   Time from screening to diagnostic mammogram, diagnostic imaging to biopsy, biopsy to pathology results known, pathology results available to when patient was informed about results, pathology known to patient to patient scheduled for consultation with a breast surgeon.

During these steps, the patient communicated with a breast-imaging scheduler, front-desk registrar, radiologist, mammography technician, and the navigator.

    Core biopsy
    Pathology results
    Patient notified
    Surgical consultation scheduled

Diagnostic evaluation and biopsy were performed on Monday, April 6. Biopsy was performed as a core biopsy in breast ultrasound. The patient was given post-procedure instructions by the mammography technician and told by the radiologist that someone will call her in a few days with the results. On Wednesday, April 8, the pathology results were available, and the patient was called by the radiologist that evening to inform her that she had invasive ductal carcinoma. The radiologist notified the ONN, who did the following:

- Informed the patient of her (the ONN's) navigation role in her care going forward, beginning with being present for her surgical consultation
- Educated the patient about the medical terms in her pathology report from the biopsy procedure
- Determined if there were any barriers preventing the patient from coming to her surgical appointment and bringing a family member or friend to accompany her
- Provided the patient an overview of what to expect during the surgical consultation

S   Schedule patient for an appointment with a breast surgeon. Note patient is a biopsy-proven-patient and should receive priority for being scheduled soon. Schedule time with the navigator to coincide with surgical consultation.

B   Identify any barriers the patient may have regarding her ability to come in for her consultation.

E   Educate patient about purpose of surgical consultation. Instruct patient to bring family member with her. Provide basic information about breast cancer diagnosis and treatment. Provide information about the role of an ONN in her care.

T   Record date results were available from pathology. Record date and time patient notified of results.

Q   Time from core biopsy to pathology results available, results available to patient being notified of pathology results, patient notified of results to patient scheduled for surgical consultation.

During these steps, the patient communicated with a breast-imaging radiologist, mammography technician, navigator, and surgical appointment scheduler.

> Breast surgical consult
> MRI
> Plastic surgery consult
> Schedule for breast cancer surgery

The patient arrives for her appointment with the breast surgeon. During the consultation, the navigator is present in the room for the clinical breast examination, review of the mammograms and ultrasounds, and discussion about the surgical treatment options. The surgeon recommends that the patient see a plastic surgeon to review her reconstruction options if she decides to have a mastectomy instead of a lumpectomy. He also requests that she be scheduled for a breast MRI: her breast tissue is very dense, and the MRI can rule out multicentric disease and confirm the size of the tumor. If lumpectomy is the option chosen (and the surgeon feels she is a good candidate for this procedure), it will be done as a wire localization procedure. The navigator did the following:

- Reiterated the information provided by the breast surgeon
- Asked the patient what milestones may be coming up in the next 6 to 9 months so they can be dovetailed with her treatment schedule
- Asked the patient what her life goals are to determine if they can prevent any phases of treatment she will be receiving from canceling them
- Explained to the patient the surgical options, wire localization procedure, survival rate statistics, and local recurrence statistics for lumpectomy versus mastectomy options
- Explained to the patient what to expect during the plastic surgery consultation
- Showed the patient photographs of the various surgical options, including lumpectomy, mastectomy, and mastectomy with various forms of reconstruction
- Assessed the patient's concerns related to intimacy and sexuality
- Provided the patient with an overview of radiation therapy treatment protocols and the necessity of radiation for women choosing lumpectomy
- Explained to the patient the breast MRI procedure, how it is done, and what information will be obtained from it that may affect decision making about surgical treatment
- Explained the sentinel node biopsy procedure and how axillary dissection is performed if the node is positive
- Assessed for barriers that may affect the patient's decision making regarding her choice of surgical options (i.e., transportation that might be needed for daily radiation therapy)
- Gave the patient educational information to take home with her as well as a list of resources pertinent to her for additional education and support

> S   Schedule patient for an appointment with a plastic surgeon in the breast center. Schedule patient for a breast MRI (factoring in her menstrual history).
>
> B   Identify any barriers the patient may have regarding coming in for her consultation or her MRI.
>
> E   Educate patient about survival stats and recurrence statistics for lumpectomy with radiation versus mastectomy. Educate patient about reconstruction options, breast MRI procedure, and sentinel node biopsy.

T   Time from request for MRI to be scheduled to MRI being performed (exclude delay due to menstrual cycle), request for plastic surgery consultation to appointment taking place.

Q   Measure patient satisfaction with surgical consultation experience, and length of time from consultation to patient being scheduled for breast cancer surgery. Measure patient satisfaction with preoperative teaching.

The patient communicated with the breast surgeon and the ONN.

Surgery procedures scheduled
Preoperative tests and H&P arranged
Preoperative teaching scheduled
Patient goes to surgery

After the MRI and consultations are completed, the navigator confirmed there were no additional findings of concern on the MRI (i.e., no multicentric disease, tumor remained same measurement) that could influence decision making about surgical options. The patient saw the plastic surgeon and discussed both implant and flap reconstruction options. The patient chose to do lumpectomy with sentinel node biopsy followed by radiation. The need for chemotherapy or hormonal therapy remains unknown for now. The operating room (OR) scheduler arranged for preoperative tests, notified the primary care provider (PCP) of the need for history & physical (H&P), and arranged the OR date and the preoperative teaching appointment. The patient had her H&P done by her PCP, along with blood work, chest X-ray, and EKG done the same day in his office on April 13. Her surgery was scheduled for April 15. The ONN did the following:

- Reviewed the results of the MRI and spoke with the surgeon to confirm that the patient remains a candidate for lumpectomy surgery if she chooses
- Reviewed the clinical note from the plastic surgeon to see the outcome of the consultation
- Contacted the patient to discuss her MRI results, her plastic surgeon consultation, and the patient's decision regarding breast surgical options
- Contacted the OR scheduler to facilitate scheduling of preoperative tests and procedures, H&P, as well as actual OR date
- Reviewed the PCP clinical notes to ensure that the patient was cleared for surgery
- Met with patient or communicated by phone to provide preoperative teaching information, including what to expect throughout her surgery day, how she might feel afterward, wound care instructions, and the necessity to have someone accompany her because she will not be allowed to drive herself home that afternoon. The sentinel node procedure was reviewed in detail because she will be receiving a radioactive isotope injection in radiology before going to the OR. The wire localization procedure was also explained in depth.
- Reviewed with patient the type of pathology information that will be learned from the surgery
- Reviewed with patient the time line for meeting with a medical oncologist and radiation oncologist, and their roles in her adjuvant therapy planning process
- Followed up on preoperative test results to ensure there were no findings that would affect surgery taking place as planned

S   Schedule preoperative tests, H&P, OR date, wire localization procedure pre-operation, sentinel node injection pre-operation, postoperative appointment 1 week following surgery, consultations post-operation with medical oncologist, consultations post-operation with radiation oncologist.

B   Assess for barriers related to preparing for surgery and immediate postoperative needs.

E   Educate patient about preoperative instructions, wound care, sentinel node biopsy procedure, possible axillary node dissection teaching, wire localization procedure, any drug administration instructions (related to her prescription and OTC drugs the patient takes on a regular basis) 24 hours prior to surgery, what to expect at time of postoperative appointment with surgeon, what to expect at time of medical and radiation oncology appointments.

T   Record the dates that following appointments were scheduled: preoperative teaching; postoperative appointments—surgical, medical oncology, and radiation oncology; and the dates they actually occurred.

Q   No delays in surgical treatment due to failure to confirm preoperative tests completed and within normal limits; patient adequately prepared by participating in preoperative teaching; MRI imaging and mammography studies correlated with one another to ensure surgical recommendations do not require changes. Measure patient satisfaction with entire treatment process to date.

Patient communicated with the navigator, surgeon, OR scheduler, PCP, pre-care nurses, OR nurses, recovery room nurses, and anesthesiology.

Discharged from ambulatory surgery recovery room
Home care
Postoperative surgical appointment

The patient's surgery is done. She underwent a wire localization lumpectomy with sentinel node biopsy. During the operation, the sentinel node was identified and sent to pathology for touch preparation analysis and results were positive for finding cancer. The patient was transferred to the recovery room. The navigator called the recovery room to get a status report on the patient. The ONN provided the recovery room nurse with information about what teaching instructions the patient had had prior to surgery. She was discharged to home with an appointment slip to return to see the surgeon in 6 days. The ONN called the patient the morning after surgery to see how she was feeling and how much drainage may be coming through her bandages. The patient returned for her postoperative appointment and was given her pathology results by the surgeon with the ONN present. Her incisions were healing well. Her tumor measured 1.4 cm of invasive ductal carcinoma. The margins were all clear for greater than 2 mm. ER was 90%; PR was 70%; HER2neu was negative; Grade 3. Ki67 was 70%. The sentinel node was positive for metastatic disease. No other nodes were removed, with the plan to have the axilla radiated. The patient was told when she would be seeing the medical oncologist and radiation oncologist and the purpose of these appointments. In preparation for the medical oncology appointment, the ONN contacted the medical oncologist to obtain information about what tests would be performed prior to the consultation.

The medical oncologist requested a CAT scan and bone scan be done, along with a MUGA scan and blood work for the purpose of conducting a staging workup. The ONN did the following:

- Ensured that the patient had clear instructions regarding her drain management and wound care at home
- Assessed her for psychosocial needs, with a focus on the new information that her sentinel node was positive
- Ensured that the patient had her postoperative appointment for surgical visit next week
- Ensured that she had contact information for medical emergencies and questions
- Reviewed the pathology report prior to the patient returning for her postoperative visit to ensure that it was available for the time of visit, what the findings were, and the completeness of the report for prognostic factors and staging information
- Joined the patient at the time of the postoperative visit with the surgeon to reiterate the findings and explain the next treatment steps
- Reviewed the schedule to ensure that the patient had information about the date, time, and location for her medical oncology and radiation oncology appointments
- Explained what to expect at the oncology appointments
- Contacted the medical oncologist to determine what staging workup tests would be desired for completion of staging information
- Explained to the patient the purpose of these tests and how it relates to planning her treatment
- Arranged for these tests to be performed

    S   Order MUGA scan, bone scan, CAT scan, blood work.

    B   Assess for any barriers that would prevent the patient from having tests and medical oncology as well as radiation oncology consultation.

    E   Educate the patient about her pathology results regarding the stage of her breast cancer, which, despite having a positive node, still had favorable prognostic factors. Educate patient about the purpose of additional tests being requested by medical oncologist in preparation for appointment.

    T   Record the dates of her medical oncology and radiation oncology appointments, and record when they were actually completed; the dates the tests that were ordered to be done and the dates when the results were back (should be prior to medical oncology consultation).

    Q   Check the completeness of pathology report, including all prognostic factors: postoperative wound infection rate, seroma rate, reexcision rate, breast conservation rate (excludes multicentric disease, inflammatory breast cancer, and/or stage III patients who had insufficient shrinkage from the neoadjuvant chemotherapy).

Patient communicated with the navigator, surgeon, recovery room nurses, and breast center nurse practitioner (NP).

Staging workup tests
Medical oncology consultation

The patient had her tests done and saw the medical oncologist the following week. Her scans were clear, with no evidence of metastasis, and her MUGA scan was within normal limits. Based on the age of the patient and her overall health, the medical oncologist recommended chemotherapy and hormonal therapy. The medical oncologist advised that specific chemotherapy drugs be given, spacing cycles 2 weeks apart, and felt she was a good candidate for the clinical trial X. The risks and benefits of treatment were reviewed in detail, and the patient agreed to participate in the clinical trial drug regimen. She received a total of 12 cycles of chemotherapy, combining a mixture of drugs over that period. She was followed closely by a medical oncology NP, who monitored her blood levels, side effects, and temperature. The ONN spoke with the patient the day after her consultation to review with her the recommendations and to address any of her questions. Because the patient had a positive sentinel node that wasn't anticipated preoperatively, the ONN scheduled her for a consultation in rehabilitation medicine with a certified lymphedema therapist. Although risk of developing lymphedema is low with the removal of just one node, this patient would be receiving additional radiation to her axilla that would increase her risk of lymphedema in the future. The patient was particularly concerned about side effects and her ability to work while receiving chemotherapy. The patient also didn't have money to purchase a wig and didn't want to start her treatment until she could afford to do so. The ONN provided her with free resources for obtaining a wig and reiterated the treatment regimen schedule and the importance of keeping her appointments with the radiation oncologist next week as well as adherence to all her chemotherapy appointments. The navigator did the following:

- Ensured that tests were performed prior to the patient seeing the medical oncologist
- Reviewed test results prior to the medical oncology appointment
- Contacted the patient one day after the medical oncology appointment to review the outcome of the visit
- Assessed the patient for possible clinical trial participation
- Provided information about chemotherapy schedules and monitoring during and between cycles
- Assessed the patient for barriers that would prevent her from adhering to therapy recommendations
- Provided the patient with contact information to obtain a free wig from the American Cancer Society and checked with her insurance company to see if it offers coverage for a skull prosthesis
- Scheduled the patient for an appointment with a certified lymphedema therapist
- Ensured that the patient has transportation for chemotherapy appointments
- Reiterated the purpose of chemotherapy and education information about the drugs and side effect management
- Confirmed that the patient has radiation oncology appointment for next week
- Assisted patient with updating her calendar with her chemotherapy treatments and home health needs

    S   Schedule chemotherapy treatment appointments every 2 weeks for 12 weeks, and schedule appointments with medical oncologist and NP alternating throughout treatment.

B   Assess for barriers that affect ability of the patient to adhere to chemotherapy regimen.

T   Record and monitor the patient's progress and compliance through chemotherapy treatment.

Q   Unplanned hospitalization during chemotherapy treatment, missed appointments for chemotherapy, adherence to National Comprehensive Cancer Network (NCCN) treatment guidelines.

The patient communicated with the ONN, medical oncologist, medical oncology NP, American Cancer Society office (for a free wig), and chemotherapy nurses.

Radiation consultation
Chemotherapy treatment
Radiation therapy treatment
Hormonal therapy treatment

The patient met with the radiation oncologist the following week for consultation and discussion about radiation therapy that will begin after completion of her chemotherapy. She was educated about the purpose of radiation and how the therapy works, as well as the schedule for radiation. She completed her chemotherapy treatment having to delay only one cycle of treatment by a week due to low blood counts. The ONN saw her during her treatment when she returned to see the surgeon 1 month and 3 months post-operation. The ONN also communicated with the patient by phone after each chemotherapy treatment and received reports from the chemotherapy nurse regarding her progress. She had one episode of nausea and vomiting that was not adequately controlled with the antiemetic drug she was given at the time of she started her initial treatment. She contacted the medical oncology doctor on call, who prescribed for her a stronger antiemetic that relieved her of her symptoms. No hospitalization was required. She was educated about radiation therapy and given literature about this type of treatment. After a 2-week break post-chemotherapy, she met with the radiation oncologist again for treatment planning. Simulation was done at the time of the first visit, and 2 days later she began her daily radiation, Monday through Friday for 6½ weeks. Other than fatigue, she did not have any concerning side effects. Upon completion of her radiation, she returned to see her medical oncologist and received information about hormonal therapy and was given a prescription to take for 5 years. She was given an appointment to see the medical oncologist again in 1 month. The navigator did the following:

- Educated the patient about chemotherapy, its side effects, and ways to reduce side effects, and monitor her health
- Educated the patient about lymphedema and ways to prevent or reduce its occurrence
- Instructed the patient about radiation therapy and the importance of adhering to the daily schedule
- Taught the patient about hormonal therapy and the importance of adhering to the daily schedule
- Assessed the patient for barriers that may affect her ability to stay on treatment regimens as prescribed
- Provided the patient with information about long-term side effects of treatment, including menopausal management caused by chemotherapy and hormonal therapy

- Ensured that the patient's appointments were scheduled at specific intervals following their departmental protocol for follow-up with the surgeon, medical oncologist, and radiation oncologist

  S   Schedule appointments for chemotherapy administration and blood work. Schedule appointments with lymphedema therapist, with the surgeon for follow-up, and for ongoing monitoring by medical oncology team and by radiation oncologist.

  B   Assess for barriers to treatment and adherence to schedule of treatment.

  E   Educate patient about chemotherapy drugs, side effects, and overall treatment schedule; radiation therapy regimen and overall treatment schedule; hormonal therapy treatment and importance of taking medication daily and consistently; potential side effects, with focus on bone health, menopausal management, and long-term side effects of chemotherapy and radiation therapy.

  T   Record test results and when they were performed, and patient's adherence to treatment schedule.

  Q   Unplanned admission to hospital during chemotherapy, unplanned breaks in radiation therapy, compliance with adherence to hormonal therapy, adherence to NCCN treatment guidelines. Measure patient satisfaction with treatment process to date.

Patient communicated with medical oncologist, radiation oncologist, navigator, NP, emergency on-call doctor, and American Cancer Society.

Completion of adjuvant therapy
Begin hormonal therapy
Long-term survivorship monitoring

The patient has completed all her therapy, with the exception of hormonal therapy. She is experiencing hot flashes and night sweats. She sees the medical oncologist 1 month after starting the medication. She complains of difficulty sleeping and feeling anxious since her chemotherapy and radiation ended. She is now seeing the surgeon every 6 months, medical oncology department every 3–4 months, and radiation oncology department every 6 months. The patient wants to have a CAT scan and bone scan repeated again and done at least annually due to fear of recurrence. The doctor told her that scans were no longer needed. The ONN did the following:

- Reiterated the importance of hormonal therapy for prevention of recurrence
- Discussed healthy lifestyle compliance to further reduce risk of recurrence
- Explained why scans are no longer routinely done post-treatment (NCCN treatment guidelines)
- Recommended that the patient attend an upcoming survivor retreat to help her with psychological issues she is experiencing, especially fear of recurrence
- Provided information and resources to help address menopausal symptoms
- Provided information regarding survivor retreats and patient educational seminars

  S   Schedule long-term follow-up appointments with each oncology discipline. Register patient for upcoming survivor retreat and education seminars for survivors. Ensure that the patient is seen annually by her PCP for a physical examination and annually by her gynecologist for a pelvic examination. Ensure that the patient is scheduled for follow-up mammogram at specific intervals, following institution's protocol for post-radiation/surgical management of breast cancer.

B   Assess for barriers to adherence to hormonal therapy and keeping future appointments.

E   Educate patient about hormonal therapy, its purpose and side effects, and control of side effects; long-term monitoring for recurrence or new onset of another cancer; lifestyle changes that can further reduce the risk of recurrence.

T   Ensure that summary information about patient's entire treatment is documented and provided to her PCP and gynecologist. Record compliance with follow-up appointments, follow-up mammograms, hormonal therapy as prescribed, lymphedema prevention methods.

Q   Measure the patient's psychological well-being at completion of treatment and transition back to PCP, outcomes of participation in survivor retreat, and survival rate.

Patient communicated with navigator and majority of her breast center team during this phase of care.

▶ Defining When Navigation Begins and Ends

When Does Navigation Start?

There are differences of opinion about when navigation starts; if you think about it, however, it should start in the local community with community outreach. This might be your responsibility or that of a patient lay navigator, a case worker, or even a social worker. The goal is to get people to come in for screenings, get diagnosed early (thus reducing the risk of getting cancer), prevent cancer altogether, undo myths, instill the facts, and remove barriers that prevent any of the above from happening.

You might be part of the team that goes into the community or you may become the navigator for newly diagnosed patients who have come in for screening and have been newly diagnosed. This type of information should be part of the chart I discussed earlier, where you record the roles and responsibilities of each member of the multidisciplinary team.

When Does Navigation End?

The point at which navigation can be unclear in some cases. Patients may have developed a dependence on you that they don't want to lose. It is important to establish guidelines; otherwise, you will find your time occupied by the "worried well" who call you for little things that take up time, for example, should the patient ask for an ultrasound when she gets her next mammogram because her cancer was found with ultrasound? Should she invest in brand-name vitamins instead of generic?

Work with your oncology team to determine the appropriate time to transition patients back to their PCPs. Some institutions have established survivorship clinics where a cancer survivor is followed long term (as in years!) by an advance practice nurse (APN). This provides patients with a lot of psychosocial support, but it may also be implying to all patients that the team who took care of them anticipates their cancer recurring when they don't at all. Some cancer centers have developed an algorithm based on risk of local recurrence and distant recurrence. For example, a patient with an early stage cancer who has a less than 10% risk of local recurrence and a 5% risk of distant recurrence should be able to be followed for one year, then transitioned to her PCP. Someone with stage 3 cancer will be best served, however, if he is followed for at least 5 years, given that these types of patients carry a much higher risk of both local and distant recurrence. It is smart to let patients know up-front, even at the time of their first consultation or postoperative appointment, how long they will be managed by the oncology team and when to plan on transitioning back to their PCP. Ideally, PCPs never become disconnected from their patients and their care. For patients with comorbidities, these diseases and disorders should still be managed by the community providers and not taken on by members of the multidisciplinary team. This is referred to as a shared-care model.

▶ Navigating Patients with Metastatic Disease

What if your patient isn't going to be a long-term survivor? Although more individuals than ever before are diagnosed with stage IV cancer and survive longer and live with their disease as a chronic illness, they can never be permanently transitioned to their community providers. With improvements in treatments, patients can live several years to possibly a decade or more, always receiving some type of treatment to control the cancer where it has spread.

The role of the ONN in these situations may be quite different from center to center. In some cases, a social worker may be assuming much of the responsibility. In others, it may be the medical oncology NP. And there are certainly many cancer centers who designate their ONNs as the primary point person for patients as they continue to be seen and treated. Ensuring that patients have resources for support, have already been seen by a palliative care provider (hopefully before symptom management becomes an issue), have information about hospice care services when appropriate, and have psychosocial support and financial resources is key. (My specialty is metastatic breast cancer so I "live" in this space.) Helping patients make decisions about their treatment options, making sure their family members have the resources they need for coping, and even helping to ensure that the patients remain in charge and are not forcefully influenced by a family member to continue treatment when they don't want to are profound roles for ONNs. They are very fulfilling roles, however. As the end of life approaches, making sure that patients have achieved all that they planned to in order to experience a good death provides me with solace because I know that I have helped these patients and their families and done the very best that I could.

▶ Summary

This chapter focused on performing operations management and correcting system problems so that you don't become a Band-Aid for a broken system. Being a Band-Aid is far less rewarding than devoting your time to what patients really need—your personal time and navigation skills as they travel through their journey. I have also provided ways that I personally evaluated how patients flowed through their breast cancer experience at Hopkins. It was eye opening for me at first and taught me to never assume anything. I have also provided tools that I used for documenting my own navigation responsibilities. I hope that you rework the case study in this chapter and apply it to your own work setting with the types of cancer patients you support or will support.

Where navigation begins and where it ends are very important points to define. There are situations in which navigators work as tandem teams, with a handoff as patients go along their journey and enter a new phase of treatment with their new ONN. The ideal situation is for patients to have the same ONN across the continuum of care.

You learned in nursing school that if you don't document it, then it wasn't done; the same applies to navigation tasks and functions. Whether you still need to use an Excel spreadsheet to track your patients or you have built into the electronic patient record a section that enables you to keep track of and share information with other members of the multidisciplinary team, you must always maintain information in the medical record as well as track statistics. Don't let data capture take a backseat. It is a vital task for you to complete. You will appreciate having this type of information later when it is time to report statistics and when you have performance evaluations done.

Next, in Chapter 5, I will tell you all about metrics.

Reference

1. Shockney L. *Becoming a Breast Cancer Nurse Navigator*. Boston, MA: Jones & Bartlett Publishing, 2011.

CHAPTER 5

Measuring the Impact That Navigation Has on Return on Investment, the Patient Experience, and Clinical Outcomes

It is not nearly sufficient to say that patients thank you for helping them navigate their cancer care. Even if you can provide individual patient anecdotes about your ability to prevent an unplanned readmission to the hospital, those involved with finance at your facility will want more statistics. Statistics that reflect the three categories of measurement stated in the title of this chapter is what is needed to demonstrate the true value of a navigation program.

The leaders of your cancer facility want to ensure that the time and money they have invested in developing and implementing your navigator role provides the intended outcomes for patients and for the cancer program as a whole. It is wonderful to have patients tell you personally how helpful you have been in navigating them through such a life-altering experience as breast cancer diagnosis and treatment. Being able to demonstrate your value to leadership is also critically important, especially in hard economic times.

In times of cost containment in the healthcare arena, being able to justify a specific program, particularly if it is new and not a billable service, is vital to the continuation of that program, including a navigation program. It is necessary to demonstrate the value of a navigation program to the overall patient care delivery system and to demonstrate that providing a coordinated navigation service enhances patient care and patient satisfaction, and results in more patients choosing to come to your breast center in the future. The following are some questions commonly asked when evaluating the success of a navigation program:[1]

- What is the effect of the patient navigator assisting patients in coordinating services, from the point of a suspicious cancer finding through noncancer resolution or cancer treatment? Include overcoming access barriers such as financial, misinformation, and healthcare system barriers.
- To what extent does the type or degree of service result in reduction and/or elimination of patient-access barriers, thereby providing more timely access to quality standard cancer care for all patients?
- To what extent does demographic matching of patient and navigator (e.g., race, ethnicity, gender) or fluency in primary language of the patient affect standard-of-care adherence and perceived satisfaction with the healthcare system?
- In terms of cost and meeting the goals of the navigation program as set forth by the breast center leadership, how effective is a patient navigator in providing patient support and assistance to eliminate patient access barriers and improve timely delivery of quality, standard cancer care?

The expectation is that navigated patients will (1) receive definitive diagnosis sooner after screening and abnormal findings, (2) receive treatments sooner after a positive diagnosis of cancer, and (3) improve their satisfaction with the healthcare system experience, and that (4) the overall result is more patients receiving appropriate treatment in keeping with National Comprehensive Cancer Network (NCCN) treatment guidelines.

Studies have been done in a variety of settings to measure scientifically how well various strategies fulfill the role of patient navigation. The questions being asked by the National Cancer Institute, who is one funder of navigation programs, include questions such as those listed above as well as the following:[1]

- Which patient navigation strategies are most effective? Those of an indigenous nonprofessional (cancer survivor, community layperson) or those of a professional healthcare provider (nurse, social worker, or other allied healthcare professional)? Volunteer navigator or paid navigator?
- Does the primary location (community-based organization, primary care screening/diagnosis clinic/center, or hospital center) of the patient navigator affect the success of the navigation?
- Does the patient navigator assisting patients in coordinating care among multiple physicians affect standard-of-care adherence and perceived satisfaction with the healthcare system?
- Does a patient navigator assisting patients through the cancer care continuum increase patients' and their families' identification and use of a usual source of care, for both cancer follow-up and other medical conditions?

To demonstrate success in answering some of these specific thought-provoking questions, you need to ensure that your breast center has in place the resources to provide the services needed. You need to document the methodologies and techniques for overcoming barriers (e.g., utilizing a primary language other than English) to timely access to cancer diagnosis and treatment services. Your breast center needs to show an adequate breast cancer screening rate. These rates ensure that a sufficient sample (based on power analysis of patients with abnormal findings) are referred to the patient navigator.

Start with collecting and recording baseline historical data and make plans for a continuous comparison group through the study period. It is important to factor in history effects, system biases, community activities that may affect changes in cancer disparities (e.g., other organizations' efforts to increase cancer screening rates) and other confounding factors.

Your needs assessment helps to determine the most frequent patient-access barriers and to identify methods and techniques to overcome these access barriers in a timely, efficient manner. You might even decide to try eliminating these barriers using several different methods and compare the methods to see which works best.

You and the oncology faculty want to establish rapport with primary care and other cancer care providers and nursing staff in your community who you anticipate working with. If you are targeting a specific neighborhood to increase mammography screening rates, reach out to the primary care physicians (PCPs) in that area as well as the community centers, churches, and other local organizations to make them aware of your intended efforts and of the goals of the program. If your focus is on increasing screening rates, you also need to know the community screening rates and number of abnormal findings currently in the cancer care continuum. Some data you need comes from Medicare information or the Medicaid database.

It is terrific when you see the community working together. You can keep records of the number of patient referrals you receive for screening mammography appointments, for example, from Dr. X (the PCP in the targeted community). This is teamwork at its best—bringing community outreach, patient navigation, and community providers together for a common goal: To increase compliance with annual mammography screening. Purchasing cab vouchers and engaging the local cab service to pick up a patient for her screening mammogram and return at a designated time to take her back home brings in other community resources that result in an increase in access to care.

Do not assume that you will remember each implementation step you have done. Record them as you implement them. Revisit your list often to see where you have been and where you still need to go. Make incremental changes. Your navigation program cannot be built in a day, not if it is to be successful.

When you are just beginning your navigation role, it can seem difficult and quite complex to figure out what measurements you want to undertake first. It is to your advantage, however, to start from the onset of the implementation of your position to measure the impact your work has on contributing to improving the delivery of patient care. Consider starting with a list of overarching goals you want to accomplish and demonstrate what your direct contribution as a nurse navigator has on breast health and breast cancer patient care. Here are areas of focus to consider when developing ways to measure specifically the value of a formal navigation program at your center:[1]

- Improved coordination of high-quality care:
  - Demonstrate that patients are not falling through the cracks as they are transitioned from one discipline (surgical oncology) to another (medical oncology and radiation oncology).
  - Demonstrate that there are no delays in providing this coordination.
- Enhanced access to services for all patients:
  - Measure the frequency of support services being used by patients (matching with a survivor volunteer for support, American Cancer Society (ACS) road to recovery, wig closet, cancer counseling center).
  - Increase the number of underserved patients having screening mammograms.

- Removal of barriers to care (track these barriers by type and record how each barrier was overcome):
  - Financial and economic
  - Language and cultural
  - Communication
  - Healthcare system
  - Transportation
  - Bias based on culture, race, or age
  - Fear
- More efficient delivery of care by measuring the time delays from one point to the next (turnaround times for results, appointment requested and appointment taking place)

■ Improved outcomes:
- Compliance with providing care that meets NCCN treatment guidelines
- Survival rates
- Stages of disease at time of diagnosis
- Adherence to treatment

■ Improved sharing of resources, such as demonstrating avoidance of rework and duplication of administrative tasks or patient education

■ Enhanced relationships with the community:
- Use of community resources
- Recruitment of patients for screening mammograms from the community through awareness efforts and events

■ Increased patient satisfaction, including specific satisfaction survey questions directed at the navigation program

■ Increased referrals of new patients to the system:
- Include the source of the referrals (patient, referring physician)
- Include the satisfaction reported by the referring physician

As you become more seasoned in your role, you will be able to advance your measurement process further to include process evaluation measures that can cover what characteristics are important to the patient navigation process. Examples include the following:

■ What services are critical to provide to the patient—for example, only overcoming cancer care access barriers or also emotional, psychological, and referral support and access for medical treatment?

■ What training and support is critical to the patient navigator—cancer prevention control, hospital procedures and administration, medical knowledge, and/or emotional and psychological support to minimize burnout? How many patients can a patient navigator effectively assist simultaneously?

■ Do other program linkages and partnerships or other agencies have an impact on the success of the patient navigation intervention strategies?

Now here is some good news to help you feel less anxious about the idea of measurements. The Academy of Oncology Nurse & Patient Navigators (AONN+) set out to create evidence-based metrics to cover these three categories because we knew that it was needed. Also, you will frequently hear me say, "You cannot manage what you do not measure." The same applies to your work as an oncology nurse navigator (ONN).

First, we knew that we needed to define the domains of knowledge that you as an ONN would need to have under your belt to be an effective ONN. These domains are listed below.

▶ AONN+ Knowledge Domains

- Community outreach and prevention
- Coordination of care/care transitions
- Patient advocacy/patient empowerment
- Psychosocial support services/assessment
- Survivorship/end of life
- Professional roles and responsibilities
- Operations management/organizational
- Development/healthcare economics
- Research/quality/performance improvement

Trust me, creating this list of knowledge domains was no simple task. It required a lot of thought, hundreds and hundreds of research articles reviewed and dissected, and then interviews with experienced ONNs about what they felt these domains should encompass. Within each domain, of course, there are specific metrics.

To give you the best look at how this process was tackled and conquered, I include in Appendix C the actual peer-reviewed article written by two of our Leadership Council members: Tricia Strusowski and Danelle Johnston. Both were key members of the Metric Task Force who, with the rest of the members of the team, accomplished this extraordinary endeavor for our AONN+ members, which I hope soon will also include you.

▶ Collecting Data Is Key to Your Success

When people look at metrics, they sometimes feel defeated before they even start. They may ask themselves, "How will I have time to collect this type of information?" "Where will it come from?" "Is it available in real time or do I have to get some data retrospectively?" There is no expectation that an ONN will collect and report on every single measure here. Thirty-five metrics is a lot.

The first step is to sit down with your supervisor. Hopefully you also have a physician champion passionate about navigation. Discuss as a team which measures have the most meaning and impact for your cancer facility. Perhaps you know there are problems with unplanned readmissions. Begin with retrospectively analyzing data from prior months and/or years that depict your baseline information. Next, determine what is needed to prevent these trips to the ER that result in hospitalization. By dissecting this information and finding the root cause, you should be able to determine what needs to be fixed. Is it a patient education issue? A family caregiver problem? A language problem? A lack of response if a patient calls the on-call telephone number? Is there a medication that could have been provided prophylactically to prevent this side effect from happening?

▶ Example of How Using Data Can Make a Difference: Case Study

I will share a story with you that happened to me when I started looking at the patient experience in the breast center 25 years ago. We had a chronic problem with patients experiencing nausea and vomiting soon after they arrived in the recovery room following mastectomy with axillary dissection surgery. As they awakened or were moved to check bandages and drains, they would complain of pain. They would be given opioids, which caused nausea, then vomiting. Vomiting pulled their chest incision and axillary incision, causing more pain. It became a catch-22 for the patient, and there seemed to be no way to break the cycle. The patient would be admitted to the hospital and this pattern continued all night into the next morning.

I personally understood the heartache of this experience for patients because 27 years ago, I was one of these patients. I recall thinking that it was bad enough to look down and see the toes on my left foot that I hadn't seen since I was 13 years old, along with the shock of my 44D breast being gone and experiencing phantom limb sensation of the breast. In addition, I experienced nausea and vomiting, which increased my pain.

We formed a multidisciplinary team to study this predicament. Initially the surgeons claimed it was the anesthesiologists' fault that the patients were throwing up. The anesthesiologists responded that the surgeons took too long to do the operation. I had to call a truce and say, "We are here for the patient. The patient awakens after losing her breast that she valued. She is scared. She doesn't know her pathology results yet. She doesn't know what other treatments she will be advised to receive. Her head is in an emesis basin, her pain is terrible, and her family is at a loss what to do. How can we make this experience easier for her?" By focusing on the patient, we made progress as a team. It took many months of tweaking and adjusting, but we decided that the patient should receive a stronger anti-emetic medication IV intraoperatively rather than waiting for her to vomit in the recovery room.

We changed the philosophy of what the operation was for. Rather than her viewing mastectomy surgery as losing something, we wanted her to see she was gaining something. (I have to credit my husband for this wisdom because this is what he told me was happening to me too.) The patient is having transformation surgery—she is being transformed from a victim into a survivor by ridding her body of the source of this disease and being carried up the survival curve while she is in the operating room. She exchanged her breast for another chance at life and that's a fair trade. When she looks down, she shouldn't focus on the idea that her breast is gone; she should see that the cancer is gone.

We then took it a step further and arranged for her to have on a surgical bra with a soft breast form in it, so when she looked down at herself her silhouette was "still whole." She would be greeted by a breast cancer survivor—whether that was myself or a survivor volunteer on our team, when she rolled into the recovery room. Her family would be brought in when she was being transitioned from the gurney to a recovery chair. This was done by walking her to the bathroom while family members were notified that they could come to the recovery room. They would literally see her walking out of the bathroom escorted by her recovery room nurse, and the family enthusiastically would say, "Look! She's up and walking!" It became a totally different experience.

Patients eventually were offered the choice of staying overnight in the hospital or going home, with a home health nurse coming to their home that night and the following morning. It wasn't long before more than 95% of our patients were saying yes to wanting to go home from the recovery room instead of spending the night in a hospital bed. And their experiences were measured, resulting in more high scores for being able to be home in their own environment, a place they had control over, while still getting their medical needs effectively addressed. Patients going home, of course, required preoperative teaching about drain care, wound care, and so on. It became empowering, however, and the patient was no longer looked upon with pity but with celebration that her primary tumor was out of her body.

I named the program "Waking Up Transformed." Our nausea rate went from 87% to 2%. And it happened because we agreed that we wanted to improve the patient's experience.

▶ Build Data Collection into Your Daily Routine

Don't look at recording information to capture in the form of statistics as an extra task. This task needs to be part of your daily routine. Don't wait until later in the week to do it either. Capture information as concurrently as you can. It must be built in and automatic instead of an afterthought. Remember, you are measuring the impact you have on patient care.

Be mindful, as I have mentioned in Chapter 3, not to take credit for improvements in care that were not related to your efforts. Give credit where credit is due.

Data are meaningful only if they will be used. Some managers have a tendency to ask navigators to collect a ton of information and then not use most of it. Collecting data just to collect data is wasted time. Consider starting with 5 metrics, and then increase the number to 10 when the first 5 have become part of your routine. See if these 10 are the most impactful.

Whenever possible, you should have retrospective data to use as baseline information; otherwise, you won't know to what degree improvements have or haven't been made. AONN+ is currently conducting a research study at several different-sized cancer centers and facilities, with a focus on a handful of metrics, capturing the data in real time within a shared database. The data collection is complete and is now being analyzed. Stay tuned for those results, which we will share at upcoming AONN+ conferences and in peer-reviewed published journals.

There is power in numbers. Don't ever doubt that. You will soon find the value of statistics and how it can change perceptions, provide accuracy about clinical outcomes, and demonstrate your worth to the multidisciplinary team.

▶ Summary

This chapter focused solely on the importance of having reliable; accurate; and, whenever possible, real-time data to demonstrate the value of oncology navigation. The metrics developed by AONN+ focuses on measuring return on investment, the patient experience, and clinical outcomes. A research study using a subset of the metrics was conducted by AONN+, and these results will be available in 2020.

In this chapter, I provided a published article from the June 2018 issue *Journal of Oncology Navigation and Survivorship*. This published article provides details about how the AONN+ metrics initiative was launched, how the 35 metrics were developed, and how each metric is mapped to a standard of care required by one or more governing bodies.

My primary message in this chapter was twofold: You cannot manage what you do not measure. You must build data collection into your daily routine.

Next, in Chapter 6, I will talk about the value of having a professional home, just for you.

Reference

1. Shockney L. *Becoming a Breast Cancer Nurse Navigator*. Sudbury, MA: Jones & Bartlett Publishers, 2011.

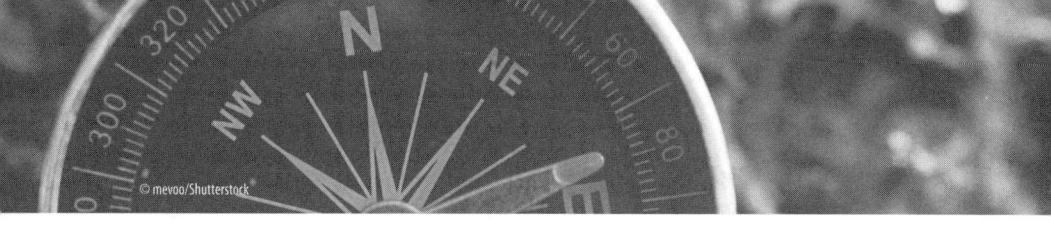

CHAPTER 6

Consider the Academy of Oncology Nurse & Patient Navigators as Your Professional Home

There may be days that you feel like you are all alone in the world of navigation. Well, you are not. There are thousands of other navigators out there, and they want to connect with you just as much as you want to connect with them.

Consider the Academy of Oncology Nurse & Patient Navigators (AONN+) to be your primary source for networking, learning, certification, training, and career advancement. It is the only national professional organization for navigation professionals and was created with you in mind.

AONN+ was founded in 2009, when nurse navigators were asking me where they could go to learn more about how to do their jobs well. Although clinical oncology nursing was where the majority of oncology nurse navigators (ONNs) were originally trained and educated to work, it was quickly recognized that this knowledge and experience would not be enough to have them become stellar ONNs. I am not the type of person to wait for someone to do something when I have already recognized the need myself and not have found resources to address the need. In collaboration with The Lynx Group, I co-founded AONN+. We began with just 96 attendees at our first conference in Baltimore, Maryland, and now the membership is almost 100 times this number. I know these numbers will keep growing because cancer facilities are either recognizing for themselves the value of navigation or they want to become accredited by the Commission on Cancer (CoC), which also requires that a navigation program be in place and effectively address the needs of the patients and community served.

AONN+ is the largest national specialty organization dedicated to improving patient care and quality of life by defining, enhancing, and promoting the role of oncology nurse and patient navigators. We are dedicated to providing a network for all professionals involved and interested in patient navigation and survivorship care services so that they can better manage the complexities of the cancer care treatment continuum for their patients. We view our organization as one consisting of "professional patient advocates" and, to that end, we support and serve our members.

▶ Mission and Vision

Mission

The mission of AONN+ is to advance the role of patient navigation in cancer care across the care continuum by providing a network for collaboration, leadership, and development of best practices for the improvement of patient access to care, evidence-based cancer treatment, and quality of life.

Vision

The vision of AONN+ is to achieve, through effective navigation, superior patient-centered quality cancer care coordination, from pre-diagnosis through survivorship and/or end of life.

Leadership Council

We have a dynamic leadership council that meets via conference call every month. The membership is diverse, with the goal of including all aspects of navigation and survivorship care. Several subcommittees focus on a specific recognized need of its membership. These needs include, but are not limited to, the areas of focus within its committees. AONN+'s committees are integral to advancing the Academy's mission and success. The current national AONN+ committees are described below.

Evidence into Practice Committee

Mission. The mission of the Evidence into Practice Committee is to bring diverse oncology professionals together to provide interactive opportunities to experience knowledge sharing, increase innovation, and enhance collaborative engagement by utilizing evidence-based practices around broad aspects of quality improvement initiatives. The Evidence into Practice Committee also strives to contribute to continued professional growth and acceleration of navigation practices.
- Abstract Review Subcommittee
- Assistance for Quality Improvement and Research (AQUIRE) Subcommittee
- Metrics Subcommittee
- Newsletter Subcommittee

Abstract Review Subcommittee
Mission. The mission of the Abstract Review Subcommittee is to review objectively AONN+ member abstracts and provide feedback for revision, with the greater goal of building momentum and evidence around navigation.

Assistance for Quality Improvement and Research (AQUIRE) Subcommittee

Mission. The mission of the AQUIRE Subcommittee is to provide mentorship support to AONN+ members in areas of quality, processes improvement, metrics, and reporting.

Metrics Subcommittee

Mission. The mission of the Metrics Subcommittee is to develop standardized metrics in the areas of return on investment, clinical outcomes, and patient experience using all the areas in which navigators practice to provide quality patient care and financial stability for their organizations.

Newsletter Subcommittee

Mission. The mission of the Newsletter Subcommittee is to produce a quarterly newsletter with a focus on providing concrete tools and resources for quality improvement, research, and metrics development that dovetails with the domains of certification for both novice and seasoned navigators.

Technology and Innovation Committee

Mission. The mission of the Technology and Innovation Committee is to focus on the use of technology to capture data and metrics for evaluation, improve quality in navigation, and provide patient education and navigator resources.

Survivorship Committee

Mission. The mission of the Survivorship Committee is to advance survivorship care throughout the continuum by providing resources and evidence-based education to clinical navigators and nonlicensed patient navigators.

Conference Planning Committee

Mission. The mission of the Conference Planning Committee is to provide relevant and high-value conference agendas and speakers that will enhance members' professional growth and development.

Clinical Trials Committee

Mission. The mission of the Clinical Trials Committee is to provide education and support to navigators to promote clinical trials to their patients and institutions.

Policy and Advocacy Committee

Mission. The mission of the Policy and Advocacy Committee is to utilize legislative, regulatory, and policy advocacy to protect and promote the practice of oncology patient navigation in order to best serve individuals and families affected by cancer.

As you can see from the above committees' focuses, we are very busy working on initiatives designed to provide you more tools, resources, and learning experiences. We also have ad hoc task forces as needed and add teams to work on specific projects.

▶ Literary Resources

The *Journal of Oncology Navigation & Survivorship* (*JONS*) is our peer-review journal for the organization. We also have *CONQUER*, which is a journal for your cancer patients. *CONQUER* is mailed to AONN+ members in a generous supply so that they are able to hand out the latest copy to their cancer patients. There is a postcard inside each journal issue that patients can complete by recording their name and address and mailing to AONN+ so that patients can continue to receive the journal delivered to their home.

I serve as chief editor for these pieces. The feedback from navigators and their patients has been overwhelmingly positive, confirming that both journals are meeting their intended needs for our membership and the patients they serve.

▶ Certification

Many of our members—both ONNs and oncology patient navigators (OPNs)—request recognition in their respective fields for being experienced oncology navigator professionals. We decided to create a certification program dedicated to the field of oncology navigation.

Prior to the article delineating roles—in *JONS* 2013;4(6):20–26—a cross matrix of AONN+, Oncology Nursing Society, and the George Washington Institute showed that clinical oncology nurses (CONs) did not coordinate at the same degree of detail, and interface with the multidisciplinary team as an ONN does. For example, most CONs coordinate care within their silos, and ONNs focus across the entire continuum. ONNs are active in and often coordinate tumor boards. Their care philosophy is based on the chronic care model, and it is driven by national guidelines like those of the National Comprehensive Cancer Network, not just chemotherapy or radiation therapy guidelines. Outreach and prevention is another area that ONNs are more involved in, and ONNs are often aware of multiple community resources, not just those that pertain to silos.

In general, *certifications can* differentiate the certified professional from other professionals *in their field*, showing that they have a demonstrated commitment to understanding and excelling in the profession. Many navigators say that the knowledge and information they gained while studying for certification provided them with ideas and strategies they had not thought of in the navigation area. Certification attests to the integrity of knowledge and skills and the reliability with which a successful certified professional can apply them. We also have in place a special certification for ONNs working with thoracic cancer patients.

AONN+ leaders have worked hard and taken the operational, legal, and financial steps needed to get our certification programs accredited. By the time you read this text, accreditation should have been achieved. The ONN general certification program Oncology Nurse Navigator-Certified General (ONN-CG) will be approved by the CoC as a recognized oncology nursing certification once accreditation is awarded. This recognition goes into effect with the CoC revised standards that begin in 2020.

▶ Annual Conferences

Two conferences are held each year. One is referred to as the midyear conference; the other is our annual national conference. Both conferences are well attended and offer a wealth of educational opportunities, networking opportunities, and examples to take home. The certification examinations are also held during this same time, occurring prior to the start of the conference itself. For May 2019, we had nearly 500 attendees for the midyear conference, which was held on the West Coast. Our national annual conference for 2019 will take place in Nashville, Tennessee, in November and will be our 10th-anniversary celebration as a nonprofit professional organization. We anticipate well over 1,000 navigators in attendance. We do our best to rotate around the country to make it as easy as possible for navigators to attend. Members have access to the presenters' slide decks. The conferences and membership are well priced to make them affordable for most.

I hope to see you at a future conference. Look for me. Tell me where you are working and how things are going in your new role as an ONN!

▶ Webinars

In recognition that not everyone can attend conferences, we offer webinars too so that learning can happen at other times.

▶ Acuity Measures

As mentioned earlier in Chapter 3, we are working on the development of an acuity tool. We believe this type of measurement will be very helpful in determining what constitutes a reasonable workload for a navigator and how specifically it was calculated.

▶ CoC Member

AONN+ became the 53rd member, out of 57, that belonged to the CoC. I serve as the CoC fellow representing you. It is refreshing to know that the CoC already created standards focused on navigation and survivorship, and welcomed us to the table to focus primarily on these two aspects of cancer care.

▶ What Would Lillie Do?

You read that right. You have the opportunity to submit questions through the AONN+ website that are sent to me regularly. I respond in real time once I receive them. I am not a wizard, but I do know a lot about the navigation field. I do my best to help you with your question or problem.

▶ Local Navigation Networks

We have local navigation networks (LNNs) and regional navigation networks who come together to meet at set intervals and listen to a speaker, have a working meeting on an initiative the members have chosen to tackle, or engage in other activities that bring together ONNs and OPNs for a common cause—navigating their patients. Some of the LNNs have even embarked on doing clinical research studies. AONN+ leadership helps an LNN get started and also provides some speaker resources periodically. Leaders of LNNs have the chance to meet with other LNN leaders when we all come together at our conferences semiannually. Soon LNNs will be able to meet virtually to avoid wide rural geographic barriers or financial costs. These local and regional networks of navigators help to facilitate communication and education among peers. We are encouraging the development of virtual networks. Currently there are over 25 LNNs.

▶ Website

The AONN+ can be reached online for more information at www.aonnonline.org. Please visit it to learn more about the organization itself. I have truly underreported all of the services and programs that are available to you. This is a great organization led by dedicated people who are passionate about oncology navigation and survivorship.

Partnerships and Other Relationships

We have various partnerships and working relationships with other professional organizations that share a common goal, striving to always provide state-of-the-art education, resources, and advances in the field of navigation and survivorship that benefit our members as well as our patients. A few of these collaborative initiatives are listed below:

- AONN+ has launched a national multisite study aimed at quantifying the value of services in terms of patient outcomes and institutions' bottom lines, a collaboration between AONN+, Chartis Oncology Solutions, LLC, and the American Cancer Society. The study has now been completed data collection, and the team is hard at work with data analytics and will be sharing preliminary study outcomes in the fall at the AONN+ national conference.
  - "By standardizing metrics under the AONN+ domains, navigators can measure the impact they have with patients from initial diagnosis to survivorship and end of life," says AONN+'s Danelle Johnston, MSN, RN, ONN-CG, OCN, Chief Nursing Officer and Senior Director of Strategic Planning and Initiatives, and a Co-Principal Investigator for the study. "These metrics are designed to be used by all organizations and programs to demonstrate the efficacy and sustainability of their programs."
  - "The data will help us produce an implementation toolkit, which other sites may use to support their efforts to track navigation metrics," says Lesley Watson, PhD, Co-Principal Investigator for the study and Principal Scientist in the Statistics and Evaluation Center at the American Cancer Society.

■ Astellas, LLC, and AONN+ are collaborating, to develop, standardize, and validate an evidence-based oncology acuity tool. When finalized, the acuity tool will be used to help oncology navigators characterize the intensity of patient navigation workload, aid in the allocation of resources, and measure the effectiveness of navigation on patient outcomes.

   • "A patient's 'acuity' refers to attributes that can be used to stratify care needs and navigation requirements," says AONN+'s Danelle Johnston, MSN, RN, ONN-CG, OCN, Chief Nursing Officer and Senior Director of Strategic Planning and Initiatives. "Once you have an accurate way to quantify and prioritize patients' needs, you can make predictions that aid in the allocation of resources."

■ Building Relationships in Delivering Genetic/Genomic Education (BRIDGE) aims to use educational interventions to best connect oncology nurses and patient navigators to cancer genetics/genomics professionals with the goal of ensuring that patients have access to the most current emerging technologies. AONN+ hopes that through this effort, patients will experience an enhanced level of care and quality of life. This project is being developed in collaboration with ISONG and the National Society of Genetic Counselors.

Literary Work

We have our own peer review journal, *JONS*, and also made a strategic decision, after being invited by the publisher, to author a textbook on navigation. It was published by Springer in 2018 titled: *Team-Based Oncology Care: The Pivotal Role of Oncology Navigation.*

■ AONN+ takes steps toward national accreditation for the ONN-CG and Oncology Patient Navigator -Certified Generalist certification examinations. The demand for certification is growing among oncology navigators; as a result, the number of people taking and passing these examinations has been steadily increasing each year.

■ The Cancer Advocacy & Patient Education Initiative (CAPE) aims to create a web-based library of best-practice information that providers in the lung cancer space can give to their patients and caregivers at each point of interaction. To develop this library, the AONN+ has partnered with Takeda Oncology and a multistakeholder coalition of leading patient advocacy organizations for lung cancer. The broader goal once CAPE-Lung is piloted is to expand this platform to other disease sites.

■ AONN+ in Partnership with Pfizer: Patient Navigation in Cancer Care 2.0 Tool kit. The tool kit examines the history and evolution of navigation, core competencies, current models of navigation, and the navigator's role along the cancer care continuum. This valuable resource, developed with the support of a dedicated Advisory Committee comprised of AONN+ leadership, explores the importance of administrative engagement and outlines standardized metrics for the development of a successful—and measurable—navigation program. The tool kit will be distributed by Pfizer through their sales and clinical educational teams. In addition, Pfizer speakers are presenting "Navigating the Cancer Care Continuum in the Context of Value-Based Cancer Care" that aligns with the tool kit, which is distributed at these talks.

- *CONQUER: the Patient Voice*: This is a journal for cancer patients and their loved ones to read and learn from, which also provides insight into how their navigators can support patients through treatment and into survivorship. Articles are written by oncology patients, sharing their stories, and also by navigators who provide information about their own professional experiences as well as tips for patients who are dealing with specific types of cancers. There are also special issues that are printed, designed to focus on specific topics, such as a specific type of cancer or a specific type of treatment modality. Members of AONN+ are shipped 25–50 copies of the journal for distribution to the patients they are currently navigating. A postcard is provided placed inside so that a patient can continue to receive future issues at home by mailing it back to our organization. This gets the patient onto our mailing list to receive the journal in their mail.

▶ Summary

This chapter has provided you an in-depth review of how the professional organization AONN+ was created with your new and future professional needs in mind, and why I recommend that you consider joining me and becoming a member. The mission and vision of AONN+, as well that of its various committees, was explained, so that you can see the depth and breadth of this organization. AONN+ and its leadership are always driven by goals and objectives that are designed to address the needs of our membership as well as the needs of oncology patients and their loved ones.

Over the last 10 years that AONN+ has existed, we have strived to listen to the needs voiced by our member. We have also worked hard to advance the field of navigation, keeping it in the forefront, so that Cancer Center Leadership as well as other professional and advocacy organizations can recognize its value and true benefits to oncology patient care.

Additional highlights about the organization were also provided, focusing on some of our partnerships, organizational relationships, and project work we are currently accomplishing.

These are exciting times for those of us in the field of oncology navigation. We will not rest on our laurels. We want to continue to provide you the professional resources, tools, and mentorship you need to be successful as an ONN.

CHAPTER 7

Where Will Your Navigation Career Take You?

Although you may be just starting out in your new role as an oncology nurse navigator (ONN), you can also begin looking into the future—your future. You may be initially filling a navigator position in a cancer facility that is relatively small, which may result in you being a generalist. This means any new cancer patient diagnosed will be seen and navigated by you. The volume of any one specific type of cancer is not large enough to warrant an ONN for organ-specific cancers in this type of setting.

You may decide, however, based on your personal interest in a specific type of cancer patient, that you want to specialize. Therefore, in a few short years, you may look at potential opportunities at a larger cancer center where organ-specific ONNs work. The most common specializations include breast, thoracic, prostate, colorectal, and gyn oncology. If this is where you see your future, then start learning as much as you can about the respective organ-specific cancer treatments. Speak with other organ-specific ONNs you meet at an Academy of Oncology Nurse & Patient Navigators (AONN+) conference. Special sessions are dedicated to high-volume, organ-specific cancers to further your focus on a specific patient population for whom you want to navigate.

If you look further down you career path, perhaps you see yourself as a nursing manager of an oncology navigation program. It is important to have an opportunity to learn more details about the tasks, functions, roles, and responsibilities for such a leader. What you see on the surface may be misleading and may not give you an accurate picture of how a nursing manager spends most of her time (and sweat). You will find some navigation job descriptions on the AONN+ website; however, no two navigators' roles and no two navigation manager jobs are identical. The organizational structure where you work (or where you will work) is different than the organizational structure at any other cancer facility. This presents an opportunity for you to learn more about the various management positions and which organizational structure you prefer. You can easily shadow another ONN who is working within an organ-specific, multidisciplinary team; however, don't anticipate getting to shadow a manager. Instead, you should be able to attend the manager track sessions at our conferences; these will give you information about the management world. You may decide, after having more information, that you don't want to go the direction you originally chose, or it may confirm for you that this is exactly the direction you want to take. Managerial roles sometimes require more formal education, for example, a master's degree in business administration (MBA). Many online colleges and universities enable people to work while going to school and avoid traveling to a university for in-person courses.

If you meet the criteria for committee participation and can devote the needed time to the committee's goals, you may be interested in getting involved in some of our committees. It is a great way to focus on clinical research, technology, survivorship, or other interests. Consider completing a performance improvement initiative or clinical research study within your clinic or oncology department: you could turn this project into a poster presentation and even possibly an oral presentation. These kinds of things will boost your résumé.

I received my registered nurse (RN) degree from a 3-year nursing diploma program based in a busy hospital. My Bachelor of Science (BS) degree is in healthcare administration. And I got my MBA from Johns Hopkins University (JHU). To explore career paths, I volunteered to do various focused projects that were recognized by senior administration at Johns Hopkins Hospital as being needed. Again, let me emphasize that I did these as a volunteer. I worked on these projects after work hours. Some projects were operations management initiatives focused, for example, on operating room throughput; others were tied to taking a closer look at the surgical oncology patient experience. This gave me great insight into whether I would enjoy each type of career move I was considering. It was common for me to be asked to fulfill a new role or expand a current role, based on having accomplished what was needed by senior administration in analyzing and studying the processes and outcomes of each project I did. You can do an online search of my name and watch a video of a presentation I did in November 2018 about my career within the field of breast cancer and the doors I opened for myself by being assertive and planning well. This presentation was the keynote speech for "A Woman's Journey" at JHU. (If you have the ebook version of this text, then click on this URL https://www.youtube.com/watch?v=JPGH4iBBeqQ&index=50.)

When I started working at Johns Hopkins in my late 20s, I never imagined that I would one day become a full professor in the JHU School of Medicine and even be appointed to a faculty chair by the medical board, president of the university, and the dean of the School of Medicine. After I had been there for about 20 years, I started to believe that it may actually be possible. I became, and currently remain, the only nurse in the country whose primary faculty appointment is in the School of Medicine and not the School of Nursing, and the only nurse without a doctorate, PhD, or MD to climb to the top of the academic ladder. When I was promoted to full professor, I was given a pin that said that I was the 226th female to become a full professor at Johns Hopkins. (My mom sent me a note that said, "I love you #226. Love, Mom." Sweet.) Just a handful of our doctors have been appointed to a physician chair as a university distinguished service professor in the last 127 years that the School of Medicine has existed and when that happened to me, I was not only thrilled but also shocked. To achieve that, you have to change clinical practice at national and international levels.

My message here is, don't ever underestimate what you can accomplish. You are your only barrier to achieving what you want to be and achieving what you want to achieve. You just need to invest yourself in your goals, work hard, and stay focused. You will need experience in each position you choose to take, so don't be in a hurry. Those who try to climb up too fast and too high can fall back down to the bottom. If you find that one type of job doesn't meet your expectations, perhaps the organizational structure, and not the job, is your barrier.

I have been at Johns Hopkins nearly 37 years, and although I am working part-time now, I continue many of my other external responsibilities, including my commitment to AONN+, public speaking, serving on medical advisory boards, and other activities. I needed to make personal decisions in 2018 about carving out more time for my family and their healthcare needs. It's all about balance.

A few years ago, I created a tree for AONN+ to use as a visual tool for helping ONNs picture where they might see themselves in 5 years, 10 years, and even 20 years from now (see **FIGURE 7-1**). Consider it a career path decision tree. Find your passion and stay the course!

You may feel so passionate about navigating individual patients across their continuum of care that you decide you never want to do anything else. That's great—because we need you!! Just be watchful of experiencing compassion fatigue and/or burnout. The next chapter focuses on preventing compassion fatigue and career burnout.

▶ Summary

My intent for this chapter was to provide you a bit more insight into my own method of evaluating possible career moves by offering my time as a volunteer first. It was and continues to be a great way to get a more candid view of what the type of roles and responsibilities might be like as well as whether I would really enjoy such a career move. Changing from one job to another is not only stressful but also exciting. And if you embark on a career change, consider offering your time as a volunteer first so that you can get a bird's-eye view of what it might look like from the inside of the organization.

A tree was also provided for you to give you some ideas about how you might create your own career path. As I mentioned in this chapter, however, if you are content doing exactly what you will be doing now—serving as an ONN for cancer patients—then don't move or change! DO, however, stay up-to-date on the methods of diagnosis, treatment modalities, survivorship care needs, and other aspects of cancer care that will enable you to always have the knowledge and expertise you need to navigate your patients well.

If you get frustrated and don't feel your voice is being heard in your current job, take advantage of one of the features of AONN+ that I referenced in Chapter 6: What would Lillie do? So what would I do in your situation? Post your question and I will personally answer you. I don't have all the answers but I usually can give you the information you need to take the next step within your workplace.

The most important message in this chapter is that you are only limited by your own beliefs of what you can and cannot accomplish. Don't let anyone tell you that you cannot accomplish something. Simply walk around them and press on…

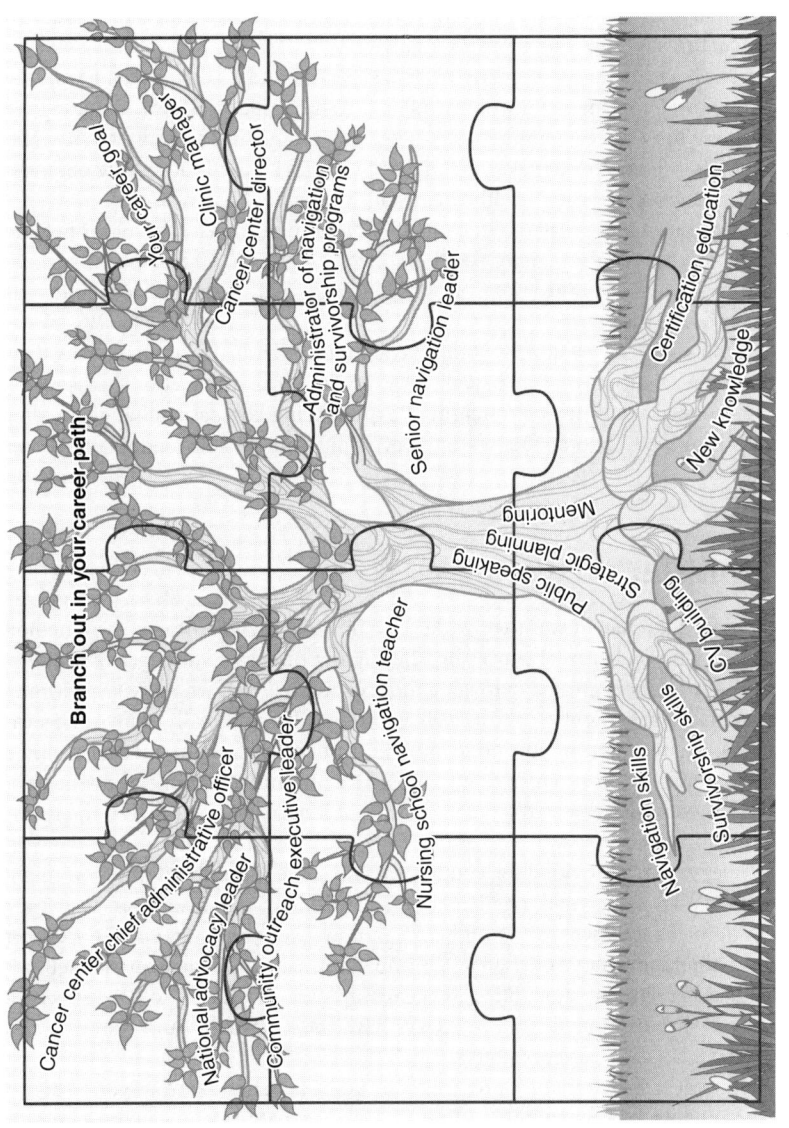

FIGURE 7-1 Branch Out in Your Career Path

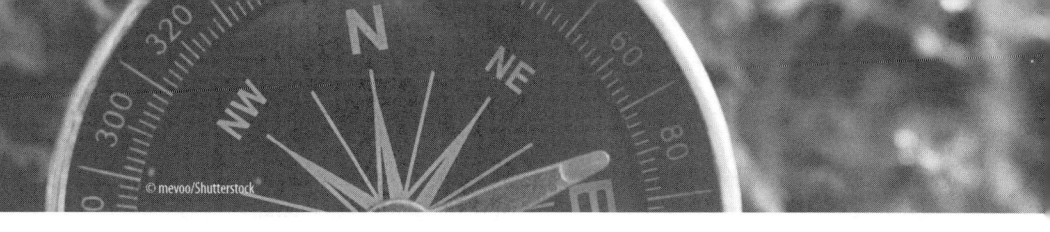

CHAPTER 8

Preventing Compassion Fatigue and Burnout

In Chapter 1 I discussed how you will be connected to patients across the continuum of care and how different that will be for you and for your patients compared to your role as a clinical oncology nurse (CON). Although it is very rewarding to have this type of role for your patients, it also means that you are a part of their lives when they are most vulnerable. You will be on this roller coaster with them when they get good news and when they get bad news. You will know your patients well because you have to know them in order to deliver patient-centered navigation. This level of continuous and long-term connection has a potential downside; however, you may experience compassion fatigue and/or burnout.

This chapter provides you with a sense of awareness, understanding, and guidance regarding how to recognize symptoms and prevent burnout as well as compassion fatigue. It contains recommendations and stress reduction resources to support you while you are caring for patients for a longer period of time, which will be different than the interval encounters you had with patients if you previously worked in an infusion center, inpatient unit, or outpatient clinic.

Now some might say that you spent a fair amount of time with your patients in these settings as well. Trust me, functioning as an oncology nurse navigator (ONN) is different. It is more engaged; it is more personal. Keep in mind that you will be helping your patients even make decisions about their treatments.

By taking care of yourself, you will be in a better position to care for your patients and address their needs. By learning about the causes and symptoms of burnout, you can take the necessary steps to prevent burnout from happening to you. Understanding and practicing ways to prevent or diminish the risk of burnout is key to your own professional survival.

▶ Defining the Terms *Compassion Fatigue* and *Burnout*[1]

Compassion fatigue is defined as a combination of secondary traumatic stress and burnout experienced by a healthcare professional providing care to others.[2]

Secondary traumatic stress is the stress that oncology professionals experience as a result of wanting to help someone who is suffering.[3] *Burnout* has been defined as accumulative stress that results in a state of physical, emotional, and mental exhaustion and occurs as a result of a person's inability to cope with the environment they are existing within.[4] In the field of oncology, burnout is manifested by a high turnover rate among oncology professionals, employee absenteeism, poor colleague support and relationships, decreased performance, a feeling of depersonalization, decreased patient satisfaction, and difficulty recruiting and retaining healthcare staff.[5]

It can be difficult to measure up to the expectations and needs of our cancer patients, especially when it comes to the level of your involvement in their lives that patients desire you to have. Burnout has been identified as one of the most common manifestations of disease among physicians, with studies specifically noting an incidence of 35% among medical oncologists, 38% among radiation oncologists, and an incidence ranging from 28% to 35% among surgical oncologists.[6] Although the average number of hours a physician works in a given week is 50, for those in the oncology field, the number is higher—63 hours per week.[7,8] No studies have been conducted looking specifically at ONNs and this work-related risk. Long hours, complex decision making for patients with life-shortening illnesses, and other issues contribute to the risk of burnout for oncology specialists. If you are now moving from an infusion center as a CON, working relatively specific and predictable hours, or soon will become an ONN, with an unpredictable work schedule, you will need to learn how to establish boundaries so that you don't make yourself continuously available to your patients. Believe me, they will expect that, particularly those who are very needy.

Burnout can happen to oncology professionals such as oncology nurses, social workers, hospice professionals, and other allied healthcare professionals. The prevalence of compassion fatigue among oncology nurses has been recorded as ranging from 8% to as high as 38%.[9] This is especially prevalent among those taking care of patients with advanced cancers. If ONNs are even more involved in the personal lives of their patients, the rate for the profession may be higher if ONNs don't take care of themselves, too.

▶ Causes of Compassion Fatigue and Burnout

A variety of contributing factors, when combined together, can cause burnout. Some specific factors warrant further discussion and understanding. Coping (or not coping) with inefficiencies within the healthcare delivery system, excess workload, loss of autonomy, and a lack of meaning in work have been identified as the primary factors.[10,11]

Growing Shortage of Oncology Specialists and Growing Volume of Cancer Patients[12]

We are entering a crisis within the oncology arena—there is a steady increase in people being diagnosed with cancer. A primary reason for this increase is the aging populating. Baby boomers are now in midlife increasing the number of people living longer. The number of people diagnosed therefore naturally increases as well.

More consumers are being screened for different types of cancer, which increases the chances of early detection. Fewer people are choosing oncology as their professional medical preference. The Institute of Medicine (IOM) predicted that by 2020, the cancer incidence will have grown by 48%, but the supply of oncologists will have increased by only 14%. There already exists a shortage of palliative care physicians, with the shortage estimated to be currently up to 7,000 (www.hhnmag .com).[13] This places a serious strain on those oncology specialists who are practicing currently and plan to continue to work in the future. The amount of time that can be spent with a patient will likely be affected by this overload of patients diagnosed in the future.

For you this means two things. You may be working with oncologists who are living in the land of compassion fatigue and burnout, perhaps making them aloof, grumpy, and seeming as if they don't care to the degree that you do about patients' emotional well-being. Because they have less time to spend with patients doing patient education, discussing treatment options in greater detail, and being more personable, you will need to fill that void for the patients you are navigating.

Inefficiencies Occurring in Multiple Directions

The prices of the newer chemotherapy and biologically targeted and personalized drugs are staggering. These drugs are under close scrutiny by third-party payers expected to cover these new and more expensive drugs. The paperwork and phone calls required to get approval for the use of these agents takes more time than it did historically. Documentation requirements associated with the decision-making process for having selected these drugs have also increased and will likely continue to do so. Clinics and consultation rooms will become more crowded with the expected continued increase in the number of people diagnosed with cancer and with no comparable increase in the number of oncology specialists to take care of them. This results in each ONN having less time to spend individual patients to address their needs and expectations. Again, you need to be the one who provides that hand to hold without letting the patient enter *your* life. You are there for them; they are not there for you.

Balancing Work and Personal Life Becomes More Complex

A study was conducted in 2008 for the purpose of evaluating the work–personal life integration among surgeons. Fifty percent reported experiencing a significant work–home life conflict, and only 36% believed that their work schedule left enough time for personal and family life.[10] Although this study was conducted with surgeons, it is an example of what can also happen to ONNs if they are not watchful of their schedules and time.

Delivering Bad News

There is no doubt that delivering bad news to patients and their loved ones can take a toll on the professional tasked with this profound responsibility. A research study conducted by Ramirez et al. demonstrated an increased rate of burnout among oncologists who felt inadequately trained in cancer communication skills. This problem carried a heavy influence on causing burn out (30% versus 17%).[14] I bring this up because, even though you may not be placed in the role of giving bad news, you will meet other ONNs who do. They are delivering the news of the pathology results from a biopsy, confirming the patient has cancer or that the cancer has spread. In some cases, this is the first encounter that an ONN has with the patient. Physicians try hard to avoid discussing how bad the bad news might be because they aren't comfortable communicating about these issues or they fear they will take away the patient's hope. This is especially prevalent with patients who are terminally ill. Studies have confirmed, however, that being honest doesn't take away hope (Smith).[15] It actually enables patients to move along the mental continuum of care so that they can realize that they will eventually succumb to this disease and need to plan for that end-of-life experience. Physician discomfort in this space is a primary reason why the average number of days a terminally ill cancer patient receives hospice care is only 5 days.

I, for reasons I may never understand, have always felt comfortable talking with patients honestly and candidly. I want them to be optimistic for as long as it is realistic, and I want to help them move along the mental continuum of care so that they go from hoping for a miracle initially to then hoping for a long life with quality that comes from living in harmony with their metastatic disease, to realizing that their life will be considerably shortened, to finally wanting to participate in the planning of experiencing a good death. Doctors are still saying to patients, "I am so sorry." Instead, I say, "I will be along your side from beginning to the end." My specialty is metastatic breast cancer patients, but I started in my twenties taking care of glioblastoma patients.

▶ The Outcome of Compassion Fatigue and Burnout

The literature suggests that the long-term effects of compassion fatigue have a negative impact on the health, work performance status, and well-being of healthcare professionals. There can be moderate to severe physical and mental health issues.[16] There can also be an increase in the use of alcohol and drugs, which may be readily accessible given the environment where healthcare professionals live and work. Feeling personal distress and angst takes a toll on anyone, but those working daily in the oncology field may be more similar to soldiers returning from war compared to others in the population. The daily assault cannot be escaped; time at home away from work is very limited; and home life, when strained, adds further to the complexities of the psychological problem. Major medical errors can and do happen, and they have been directly correlated with symptoms of burnout.[11] With the challenge of taking care of more patients with fewer doctors and nurses to manage their care, the outcomes can be devastating for all—oncology specialists, patients, and caregivers.

▶ Preventing and Recovering from Burnout

One of the best ways oncology professionals can help themselves is by taking the advice that they give to their patients: Live a healthy lifestyle, including a healthy nutritious diet; exercise; adequate sleep; stress management; committing to family time; and committing to social time, which might be church, or socializing with others over a meal. No matter how difficult this may be, work–personal life balance is still needed, and you need to make a commitment to it. I always ask my patients what gives them joy. We need to ask ourselves the same question. Delaying joy means missing a part of your life that is important to experience and cherish. Qualitative research has demonstrated that physicians who find meaning in work incorporate a philosophy of work–personal life balance and focus on what they value most.[6,17,18]

Talking with peers about what we are struggling with is therapeutic as long as it isn't a chronic complaining type of discussion. If someone you work with and admire seems to have figured out a work–personal life balance, ask them what he or she did to create it. Don't assume someone who seems to have it all together actually has it all together, and don't assume that they have less work than you. Even taking an online course on time management might enlighten you to new and innovative ways to work more efficiently, know what to delegate and to whom, and manage your personal time and optimize it. A strategy that may work for one person may not work for another, so we owe it to ourselves, our family, and our patients to commit to creating a more workable schedule that enables good patient care while simultaneously provides quality time for us outside the medical setting. Research has also validated that training healthcare professionals in mindfulness and learning techniques to improve self-awareness results in a reduction in burnout and improvements in empathy.[19]

We also know that feeling a sense of purpose and meaning in our work has to be present in order to reduce the risk of burnout and achieve a sense of life satisfaction.[1,20] If we are successful in supporting and guiding our patients, as they deserve to be, then we can feel fulfilled we are doing our job well. We can provide them with information so they can participate more confidently in the decision making about their treatment and care that fulfills their personal goals. We can feel a sense of accomplishment when our patients meet their goals. For those patients with advanced disease, we can also reminisce about the hopes the patient and family members had and how we helped them transition through various phases of hope to reaching a point of acceptance of their impending death.

To derive meaning from our work, we must identify professional values, goals, and motivators, followed by a plan to work on these specific areas. Our relationship with our patients and coworkers, the research we do to improve care for future patients, and the teaching we provide to mentor future clinicians needs to be the actual foundation that provides us with meaning as oncology professionals.[21]

Methods to prevent burnout include programs on resiliency training. These programs were specifically designed to educate participants about compassion fatigue, factors that cause chronic stress, the impact of chronic sympathetic stimulation on cognitive and behavioral function, and developing an understanding of the importance of practicing stress management on the job.[22]

Successful strategies are designed to either increase our awareness or to reduce the high level of negative arousal that characterizes stress. Techniques that have proven beneficial include relaxation techniques; promotion of healthy lifestyles, including physical training; and cognitive behavioral techniques, such as behavioral rehearsal. Cognitive behavioral techniques are particularly important because burnout often includes unrealistic expectations and false hopes.[22]

Care for the Professional Caregiver Program has proven helpful for preventing burnout. It was developed by Wellspring, which is a network of community support centers for cancer patients. Its mission is to address issues unique to professionals while providing care to patients who are very ill and dying. Although originally developed for oncology nurses, Wellspring has expanded the program for all oncology professionals. It provides interventions that support oncology team members with adaptive coping with grief, understanding the components of burnout, and demonstrations of self-care strategies to reduce workplace stressors.[23]

Stress management training through the use of technology can also prevent burnout. Research studies have demonstrated that watching video clips on a mobile device of a garden, a lake, or a waterfall can provide a sense of calm and reduce anxiety.[24]

▶ Basic Strategies That Are Beneficial for Oncology Professionals[1]

Keep Family Members Close

Carrying a cell phone or other technology enables us to send and receive quick messages or photos from our family each day. Just having a recording on your phone of your toddler laughing can soothe a distressed body and mind.

Practice Mindfulness

Take 5 minutes and go to a quiet spot and be in the moment. Look at your surroundings and relate to them. It could be a nature setting or the architecture of a building, or watching children playing on a playground. These kinds of activities pull you away from the chaos and into a quiet zone that provides a few minutes of respite. They can also be combined with mindful breathing.

Perform Operations Management of Your Workday

Identify issues that waste time or require rework; find ways to avoid them in an objective and thoughtful manner. All medical institutions are interested in hearing ways to improve efficiency because inefficiency costs money. But remember, I don't want you serving as a Band-Aid for a broken system.

Eat Healthy Meals

It can be easy to grab a soda and chips, but it is better to eat a protein bar with a glass of water. Plan balanced meals for the rest of your meals.

Traveling to and from Work

Soothing music on a CD player in your car or paying attention to scenery while staying mindful about the traffic is helpful. If you have access to public transportation, consider trying it. A bus or subway ride might provide additional time for meditation, reading, or catching up with emails. Public transportation removes you from the worries of driving in traffic, which can produce stress.

Massage

Professional massage may not be practical or affordable, but if you have a partner, the two of you can provide this to one another. Re-create a spa environment, with soft lights, soft music, scented candles, and scented oils.

Keep a Journal

Keeping a journal doesn't require writing pages of text every night. You may write just a few words that sum up your day. Expand on the topic if it was something that made you feel really good, really happy. Record these in your favorite color so they are easy to find. Time passes and we forget the good things. Recording them and making them easy to spot within a journal can provide a moment to relive and reflect on that joy.

Laughter Is Powerful Medicine

Laughter is one of the best stress relievers. If you can't find anything to laugh about, go online and find websites that feature jokes. YouTube is a good option. Three or four minutes of amusing distraction from your workday can allow you to return to your duties feeling a little better.

Employee Assistance

Most institutions offer employee assistance programs designed to provide confidential and professional support during difficult times. Psychologists and psychotherapists can be very helpful in giving perspective and advice and serving as a sounding board, especially if you prefer not to disclose your compassion fatigue and burnout symptoms to your colleagues.

Perfection Is Not the Goal

No one is saying that you need to be Wonder Woman for your patients. Ask your spouse or other loved ones to take on some tasks at home. This will give you more time with family.

Focus on What You Can Do, Not on What You Can't

We ask our patients to focus on what they can still do and less on what they are no longer able to do, and we should ask the same of ourselves. We aren't able to save the lives of our patients with terminally ill cancers. We are able to orchestrate a good death. Reflect on the positive accomplishments for your patients rather than on the negative ones. Keep your own glass half full and not half empty.

Music

Meditate or dance to music. Getting your body moving is good exercise and a stress reliever unto itself. Listening to music can be a great escape.

▶ Summary

Burnout is a reality that we must recognize in order to prevent it. Oncology is a field known for burnout. Dealing daily with life and death (and, for some of us, more death than life) can result in frustration and sadness. If we are also facing inefficient clinical operations within our work environment and other demands on our time, including family concerns, we can feel like the days are blending into one another. We tell our patients to make each day count and to participate in activities that bring joy to their lives, but we often do not abide by the same good advice. We can plan our schedules to factor in even 10-minute meditation sessions during our workday, or we can plan a vacation in advance with coverage from colleagues to look after our patients while we are away getting rejuvenated.

Being aware of the causes of burnout and compassion fatigue is the first step in diminishing their effects. Some of the factors include less-than-adequate institutional infrastructure; the demands of insurance companies; inability to find an effective work–personal life balance; and, last but certainly not least, the potential necessity to be the person to deliver bad news to our patients and their loved ones.

There are known warning signs of impending burnout. Signs include being emotionally exhausted most of the time, acting like a cynic, feeling ineffective at doing our job, and feeling a lack of personal accomplishment related to our work. There are also methods and activities available to help reduce or even prevent burnout. It is an ONN's responsibility to acknowledge the symptoms and follow interventions to prevent burnout.

One of the most important things that we do for our patients is orchestrating a good death for them. This task can allow ONNs to reap incredible benefits and satisfaction. Reflect on those patients who experienced no pain and died peacefully, had their affairs in order prior to their death, felt and knew their sense of purpose in having lived, and participated actively and confidently in the decision making about their treatment and care. These are tremendous gifts that ONNs give to their patients. Their work also reaffirms perhaps their own purpose in life—to provide end-of-life gifts that preserve the spirit and soul.

References

1. Shockney L. *Fulfilling Hope: Supporting the Needs of Advanced Cancer Patients*. New York, NY: Nova Science, 2014.
2. Figley CR. *Compassion Fatigue: Coping with Secondary Traumatic Stress Disorder in Those Who Treat the Traumatized*. New York, NY: Brunner/Mazel, 1995.
3. Figley CR. Compassion fatigue: Toward a new understanding of the costs of caring. In BH Stamm (Ed.), *Secondary Traumatic Stress: Self-Care Issues for Clinicians, Researchers, and Educators*, 2nd ed. Lutherville, MD: Sidran, 1999, 3–28.
4. Maslach C. *Burnout: The Cost of Caring*. Englewood Cliffs, NJ: Prentice-Hall, 1982.
5. Vahey DC, Aiken LH, Sloane DM, et al. Nurse burnout and patient satisfaction. *Med Care*. 2004;42(2, Suppl):II57–II66.
6. Shanafelt TD, Dyrbye L. Oncologist burnout: Causes, consequences, and responses. *J Clin Oncol*. 2012;30:1235–1241.
7. Staiger DO, Auerbach DI, Buerhaus PI. Trends in the work hours of physicians in the United States. *JAMA*. 2010;303:747–753.
8. Wetterneck TB, Linzer M, McMurray JE, et al. Work life and satisfaction of general internists. *Arch Intern Med*. 2002;162:649–656.

9. Potter P, Deshields T, Divanbeigi J, et al. Compassion fatigue and burnout: Prevalence among oncology nurses [Online exclusive]. *CJON*. 2010;14:E56–E62.

10. Shanafelt TD, Balch CM, Bechamps GJ, et al. Burnout and career satisfaction among American surgeons. *Ann Surg*. 2009;250:463–471.

11. Shanafelt TD, Balch CM, Bechamps GJ, et al. Burnout and career satisfaction among American surgeons. *Ann Surg*. 2010;251:995–1000.

12. IOM Report. *From Cancer Patient to Cancer Survivor: Lost in Transition*. 2005 http://www .nationalacademies.org/hmd/Reports/2005/From-Cancer-Patient-to-Cancer-Survivor-Lost -in-Transition.aspx. Accessed May 8, 2019.

13. www.hhnmag.com. Accessed July 22, 2019.

14. Ramirez AJ, Graham J, Richards MA, et al. Burnout and psychiatric disorder among cancer clinicians. *Br J Cancer*. 1995;71:1263–1269.

15. Smith TJ, Dow LA, Virago E, Khatcheressian J, Lyckholm LJ, Matsuyama R. Giving honest information to patients with advanced cancer maintains hope. *Oncology (Williston Park)*. 2010;24(6):521–525.

16. Stamm BH. Measuring compassion satisfaction as well as fatigue: Developmental history of the compassion satisfaction and fatigue test. In CR Figley (Ed.), *Treating Compassion Fatigue*. New York, NY: Brunner-Routledge, 2002, 107-119.

17. Shanafelt TD, Chung H, White H, et al. Shaping your career to maximize personal satisfaction in the practice of oncology. *J Clin Oncol*. 2006;24:4020–4026.

18. Shanafelt TD, Novotny P, Johnson ME, et al. The well-being and personal wellness promotion strategies of medical oncologists in the North Center Cancer Treatment Group. *Oncology*. 2005;68:23–32.

19. Epstein RM. Mindful practice. *JAMA*. 1999;282:833–839.

20. Back AL, Deignan PF, Potter PA. Compassion, compassion fatigue, and burnout: Key insights for oncology professionals. *Am Soc Clin Oncol Educ Book*. 2014:e454–e459.

21. McMurray JE, Linzer M, Konrad TR, et al. The work lives of women physicians. *J Gen Intern Med*. 2000;15(6):372–380.

22. Gentry JE. Compassion fatigue: A crucible of transformation. *J Trauma Pract*. 2002;1(3–4):37–61.

23. Shanafelt TD, Sloan JA, Habermann TM. The well-being of physicians. *Am J Med*. 2003; 114:513–519.

24. Edmonds C, Lockwood GM, Bezjak A. Alleviating emotional exhaustion in oncology nurses: An evaluation of Wellspring's Care for the Professional Caregiver Program. *J Canc Educ*. 2012; 27:27–36.

25. Villani D, Grassi A, Cognetta C, et al. The effects of a mobile stress management protocol on nurses working with cancer patients: Preliminary controlled study. *Psychol Serv*. 2013; 10(3):315–322.

Appendix A

Overview of Professional Roles and Responsibilities

The guiding principles of patient navigation are to ensure that quality, confidentiality, and professionalism are threaded throughout all aspects of care and programming.[1] Inherent in the process is continuous quality care for patients, from screening through diagnosis and treatment, based on the following tenets:

- Culturally competent care
- Confidentiality
- Respect
- Compassion
- Patient safety

Visit the AONN+ website at https://aonnonline.org/education/learning-guides /22-learning-guide-professional-roles-and-responsibilities for more information about how to apply the learning principles needed to navigate your cancer patients effectively.

▶ Roles and Responsibilities

This overview of the patient flow through the system of care defines the point at which navigation begins and the point at which navigation ends. These are a fundamental principle of navigation, as is "patient navigation should be defined with a clear scope of practice that distinguishes the role and responsibilities of the navigator from that of all other providers."[2] Blaseg points out that a clear scope of practice with stop and start points will prevent overlap of the roles of others.[3] If this fundamental point is ignored in haste to initiate a navigation program and tasks are assigned to ensure a sense of productivity and value with the role, two things can occur: (1) the navigator can assume responsibility for the role of others and (2) any difficulties associated with an individual patient's circumstances can be deferred to the navigator. This can create team difficulty and frustration to the navigator, who becomes the perennial go-to for patient problems.

Once role boundaries are defined, common responsibilities of a nurse navigator may include:

- Providing education and support to the patient and family

- Identifying special needs of the patient and delegating to appropriate support staff members
- Enhancing understanding of treatment options available
- Facilitating patient care plan recommendations by physician
- Connecting patient and family with community resources
- Coordinating multidisciplinary care from time of diagnosis throughout treatment
- Improving timeliness of appointments
- Serving as a resource for the community on health issues, prevention, screening, treatment, and research

Confusion can exist about the navigator role and responsibility. Nurse navigators commonly spend time doing clerical tasks such as faxing documents, waiting on the phone for precertification, and scheduling appointments for patients. This time is best spent *with* patients in education, psychosocial counseling, or facilitating multidisciplinary care. On the AONN+ website, the definition of navigators describes this distinction.[4] Willis and colleagues published research about a collaborative project with national stakeholders in navigation to create a role delineation framework.[5] The final framework is composed of 12 functional domains, with differences between community health workers, patient navigators, and clinically licensed navigators described in each frame.

The annual evaluation of the patient navigation process outcomes is the primary element in the American College of Surgeons Commission on Cancer (CoC) Standard 3.1: Patient Navigation Process that will influence modifications to the nurse navigator's process of care. The patient navigation process, driven by a community needs assessment, is established to address healthcare disparities and barriers to care for patients. Resources to address identified barriers may be provided either onsite or by referral to community-based or national organizations. The intent of the standard is to identify and address a new barrier each year. However, programs are allowed to address the same barrier or disparity for more than 1 year if the cancer committee documents in their minutes that they have put forth significant activity over the year but that the need to address that barrier is ongoing. The cancer committee may decide to continue work to address the barrier until the issue is resolved, for a period not to exceed 3 years between CoC program surveys.

Skills such as advocacy, problem solving, time management, critical thinking, multitasking, collaboration, and communication were identified in the Oncology Nursing Society oncology nurse navigation role delineation study.[6] AONN+ has identified additional skills of leadership and systems management. Leadership skills of the nurse navigator are expressed in several publications, and the role is depicted as one that often survives in a macro-managed environment—a role that needs minimal supervision. Seek and Hogle stressed this skill as the navigator works through the complex healthcare system to coordinate optimal care.[7] Blaseg describes it as a desired quality for a nurse navigator—one who can make decisions and work independently within the bounds of the role and demonstrate personal and professional accountability with a commitment to lifelong learning.[3] According to Vargas and colleagues, they remain flexible to possibilities of care.[8] Systems management is best described by Fillion and colleagues, who wrote that the workflow of nurse navigation is two-dimensional: patient-centered and health system–oriented.[9] Doll and colleagues state that nurse navigators possess oversight of the comprehensive care needs; provide education and advocacy for the patient; link the patient to networks of professional and community resources; and act as a distinct, constant contact to enhance psychosocial care.[10] Blaseg describes the nurse navigator's knowledge of resources as comprehensive across the healthcare system, community, and population served.[3] An example of this systemic overview is shown in the work by Christensen and Bellomo with the navigation process that demonstrated a decrease in system time as well as a cost advantage to the healthcare system.[11]

The Oncology Nursing Society[12] further defines the nurse navigator professional role as one of lifelong learning and evidence-based practice. The society encourages contribution to the knowledge base of the profession. The nurse navigator is expected to contribute to program development; participate in ethical decision making for patients; and collaborate with the cancer committee, administration, and healthcare team members.

References

1. Freeman HP. A model patient navigator program. *Oncol Issues*. 2004;19:44–46.
2. Freeman H, Rodriguez RL. History and principles of patient navigation. *Cancer*. 2011;117: 3539–3542.
3. Blaseg K. Getting started as a nurse navigator. In: Blaseg K, Daugherty P, Gamblin K, eds. *Oncology Nurse Navigation Delivering Patient-Centered Care Across the Continuum*. Pittsburgh, PA: Oncology Nursing Society, 2014, 20–42.
4. AONN+ website. FAQ. What is the difference between a nurse navigator and a patient navigator? www.aonnonline.org/about/faq. Accessed April 11, 2019.
5. Willis A, Reed E, Pratt-Chapman M, et al. Development of a framework for patient navigation: Delineating roles across navigator types. *J Oncol Navig Surviv*. 2013;4(6):20–26.
6. Brown CG, Cantril C, McMullen L, et al. Oncology nurse navigator role delineation study: An Oncology Nursing Society report. *Clin J Oncol Nurs*. 2012;16:581–585.
7. Seek A, Hogle W. Modeling a better way: Navigating the healthcare system for patients with lung cancer. *Clin J Oncol Nurs*. 2007;11:81–85.
8. Vargas RB, Ryan GW, Jackson CA, et al. Characteristics of the original patient navigation programs to reduce disparities in the diagnosis and treatment of breast cancer. *Cancer*. 2008;113:426–433.
9. Fillion L, Cook S, Veillette A, et al. Professional navigation framework: Elaboration and validation in a Canadian context. *Oncol Nurs Forum*. 2012;39:E58–E69.
10. Doll R, Barroetavena MC, Ellwood AL, et al. The cancer care navigator: Toward a conceptual framework for a new role in oncology. *Oncol Exchange*. 2007;6(4):28–33.
11. Christensen D, Bellomo C. Using a nurse navigation pathway in the timely care of oncology patients. *J Oncol Navig Surviv*. 2014;5(3):13–18.
12. Oncology Nursing Society. Oncology nurse navigator core competencies. www.ons.org/sites /default/files/ONNCompetencies_rev.pdf. Accessed April 11, 2019.

Additional Reading

Accreditation Committee Clarifications for Standards 3.1: Patient Navigation Process and 3.2: Psychosocial Distress Screening. www.facs.org/publications/newsletters/coc-source/special -source/standard3132.
American Nurses Association. Code of ethics for nurses with interpretive statements. http://www .nursingworld.org/MainMenuCategories/EthicsStandards/CodeofEthicsforNurses/Code-of -Ethics-For-Nurses.html.
Braun K, Kagawa-Singer M, Holden A, et al. Cancer patient navigator tasks across the cancer care continuum. *J Health Care Poor Underserv*. 2012;23:398–413.
Case MA. Oncology nurse navigator. *Clin J Oncol Nurs*. 2011;15:33–40.

Espinosa AR, Gabel M, Vlahakis P. Patient navigation: Defining metrics that support and justify the nurse navigator position. *J Oncol Navig Surviv*. 2012;3(5):16–20.

Fiscella K, Ransom S, Jean-Pierre P, et al. Patient-reported outcome measures suitable to assessment of patient navigation. *Cancer*. 2011;117:3603–3617.

Gentry SS, Sellers JB. Navigation considerations when working with patients. In: Blaseg K, Daugherty P, Gamblin K, eds. *Oncology Nurse Navigation: Delivering Patient-Centered Care Across the Continuum*. Pittsburgh, PA: Oncology Nursing Society, 2014:71–120.

George Washington Cancer Institute Online Academy. http://smhs.gwu.edu/gwci/education. Accessed April 11, 2019.

Johnston D. Current state of care transitions and cancer survivorship. *J Oncol Navig Surviv*. 2013;4(4):11–20.

Mack NA, Shalkowski L. How to start and expand a nurse navigation program. In: Blaseg K, Daugherty P, Gamblin K, eds. *Oncology Nurse Navigation Delivering Patient-Centered Care Across the Continuum*. Pittsburgh, PA: Oncology Nursing Society, 2014, 43–70.

Sein E. What is the patient navigator role in oncology quality metrics? www.aonnonline.org /education/interactive-learning/. Accessed June 12, 2016.

Shockney L. *Becoming a Breast Cancer Nurse Navigator*. 1st ed. Sudbury, MA: Jones and Bartlett Publishers, 2010.

Shockney L. Evolution of patient navigation. *Clin J Oncol Nurs*. 2014, 405–407.

Appendix B

Community Outreach and Prevention

Navigation is an important aspect of oncology care. The National Cancer Institute Center for Health Disparities defines patient navigation as follows: "Patient navigation refers to support and guidance offered to persons with an abnormal cancer screening or a new cancer diagnosis in accessing the cancer care system, overcoming barriers, and facilitating timely, quality care provided in a culturally sensitive manner. Patient navigation is intended to target those who are most at risk for delays in care, including racial and ethnic minorities and those from low-income populations. Furthermore, patient navigation targets specific time points in the cancer care continuum; we operationally define patient navigation as starting at the time of an abnormal screening result and ending at the determination that the screening test was a false positive or, for those individuals with a new cancer diagnosis, continuing through the completion of cancer treatment. The goal of patient navigation is to facilitate timely access to quality cancer care that meets cultural needs and standards of care for all patients."[1]

Patient navigation is recognized by the Commission on Cancer (CoC) as an essential component of oncology care. CoC organizations are mandated to have navigation in place and be able to speak to the standard at the time of survey. CoC Standard 3.1, which refers to patient navigation, states: "Patient navigation in cancer care refers to specialized assistance for the community, patients, families, and caregivers to assist in overcoming barriers to receiving care and facilitating timely access to clinical services and resources."[2] Resources identified may be provided onsite or by referral. Program evaluation is done yearly and reported to the cancer committee. Processes are modified or enhanced each year to address additional barriers identified by the community needs assessment (CNA).

Each navigation program is unique because it is based on the results of the CNA done by the organization or community that identifies the disparities and barriers that patients face. The navigation process is modified or enhanced each year to address additional barriers identified by the CNA. The CNA identifies barriers to care in the community and allows for the development of programs and community outreach events to decrease identified barriers. It also highlights issues related to access to care. A CNA is done every 3 years, and the navigation program is established and then changed to meet the needs identified.[3]

The Healthy People 2020 initiative identifies topics considered to be social determinants of health and identifies goals to improve healthcare, which include improving access to care and decreasing disparities. The four components of access to care are coverage, services, timeliness, and workforce. Access to health services is essential as disparities in access to health services affect individuals and society and lead to delays in care, lack of preventive services, hospitalizations that could have been avoided, and unmet health needs.[4] Access to healthcare has an impact on the following:

- Overall physical, social, and mental health status
- Prevention of disease and disability
- Detection and treatment of health conditions
- Quality of life
- Preventable death

Healthcare today is very complex. It is becoming increasingly difficult for patients to obtain timely care and become connected to the resources they need. One of the hats that navigators wear is that of helping to decrease barriers to care, identifying resources that will help the patient through the course of treatment, and ensuring that patients get the recommended screenings needed to stay healthy. Goals of navigation include targeting those populations with the greatest needs, decreasing barriers to care, and improving access to the healthcare system with the goal of improving timely high-quality care along with improved outcomes.

The navigation process assists patients throughout the cancer care continuum, which progresses from pre-diagnosis or diagnosis to treatment, to post-treatment and survivorship, to end-of-life care. Although there is no consensus around an optimal point for the patient's entry into patient navigation in the cancer continuum, the patient–navigator relationship begins at the initial contact with the patient. Early contact with the patient is important for establishing a relationship with the patient. However, the navigator could enter into the continuum at any point, depending on the scope of the program at each institution.[5]

There are many components to navigation. This appendix focuses on community outreach, which includes prevention and screening.

Patients face many barriers to care, which can be broken down to the following areas:

- Logistical
- Financial
- Treatment
- Social
- Communication
- Emotional/physical health

Logistical barriers include transportation issues, distance from the cancer center, lack of family and/or social support, poor care coordination, and multiple appointments at different locations. Resources vary throughout the United States, so it is important that the navigator know about local resources. Navigators can assist with troubleshooting resources and developing a transportation plan to help the patient move back and forth to treatment. Resources for transportation include the following:

- Local American Cancer Society programs
- Community transit systems
- Public transportation services

- Private services
- Some Medicaid plans may provide transportation assistance
- Charity Air flights
- Friends, family, and community resources

The Affordable Care Act has expanded insurance coverage and helped to remove barriers to care by obtaining insurance coverage for previously uninsured patients, prohibiting the denial of insurance to people with preexisting conditions, extending dependent coverage, and requiring insurance providers to cover cancer screening.[6] According to "Cancer Facts & Figures 2015," one in five people with health insurance who are diagnosed with cancer use all or most of their savings because of the financial cost of dealing with cancer. Patients who have no insurance or who are underinsured have higher medical costs, poorer outcomes, and higher rates of death.[7]

Financial toxicity is a huge barrier for cancer patients and often affects a patient's decision to stay on treatment. Financial toxicity refers to the way out-of-pocket expenses can drain the wallets of cancer patients, affect quality of life, and in fact become an adverse event of treatment. Patients often face high co-pays both for clinic visits and medications; face job loss as a result of their diagnosis and treatment; and are unable to meet their financial obligations such as rent, food, and other monthly bills. In addition, many patients have low socioeconomic status, which affects their ability to meet basic needs. If a cancer center has a financial advocate, an appointment should be scheduled so that patients can meet the advocate at their first clinic visit. Financial resources include the following:

- Disease-specific organizations
- Cancer care
- Charity care at the point of care
- Financial advocate if available
- Pharmaceutical companies and specialty pharmacies
- American Cancer Society
- Chronic Disease Fund
- Patient Access Network
- Vocational rehabilitation
- Local charitable organizations

The navigator can assist patients in overcoming treatment barriers by connecting patients with disease-specific organizations such as Support for People with Oral and Head and Neck Cancer or the Multiple Myeloma Research Foundation. Providing patient education and support is a large part of the navigator's role.

Education regarding treatment and side effects can help patients better understand their treatment and be more compliant in care. It is important to ascertain the patient's goals of care and how a navigator can advocate for the patient and support those goals. This is especially true because their goals may not be congruent with those of the healthcare team. Compliance issues may arise when these goals are not aligned.

Treatment-related toxicities are often reasons that patients do not adhere to the prescribed plan of care. Patients often give up on treatment due to the side effects that affect their quality of life. Navigators play a key role by addressing patients' concerns and making sure that the team is aware of patients' side effects. Ensuring that patients are connected with the proper resources during treatment, such as a pharmacist, a nutritionist, and a supportive care team, can help the patient make it through treatment. Treatment barriers may include the following:

- Lack of adherence to prescribed regimen, especially oral oncolytics
- Treatment side effects
- Lifestyle and habits
- Complacency
- Lack of understanding of treatment plan
- Patients lost to follow-up care

Emotional and social barriers can manifest in many ways. Social and emotional barriers that impede care may include the following: age, comorbidities, sensory changes, environmental factors (smoking, alcohol use), lack of family and/or social support, poor family dynamics, mental health issues, and living conditions. As navigators, it is important to realize that we cannot change family dynamics, but we can try to connect patients with resources to live a healthier lifestyle, such as smoking cessation programs, counseling, and community resources for drug and alcohol abuse, and assisting them with finding a primary care provider to follow them in survivorship care. Other ancillary services, such as nutrition; physical therapy; mental health counseling;, occupational therapy; and integrative therapies such as acupuncture, reiki, and massage, may help in obtaining a healthy lifestyle as well as helping mange the side effects of treatment. Providing calendars and written material at the appropriate literacy level and in patients' language are useful tools to help patients.

It is important to remember the caregiver(s) in the treatment plan. Caregiving is not easy, and many caregivers get overwhelmed. They will need additional support as well. Resources for caregivers include counseling, support groups, respite care, and the cancer center social worker.

Spiritual distress is a disruption of a person's belief or value system that can occur at any time in the disease course. It often surfaces at a time of stress, and it is important for the navigator to identify and understand cultural norms related to patients' health and illness. Healthcare providers need to ensure that their beliefs and values do not interfere with care. Resources for spiritual distress include the following: The pastoral care department, if one is available; local clergy; and the patient's clergy and support system.

Communication barriers come in many forms, such as speaking a different language, sensory changes such as visual or hearing loss, cognitive loss, and literacy issues. Patients are often confused about tests, medication administration, appointments, and the treatment plan. Navigators can assist in eliminating communication barriers by using translation services and providing educational materials in the patient's language that is culturally sensitive and at the appropriate literacy level. Communication must be assessed at each patient interaction to evaluate the patent's understanding of the disease and treatment, as well as to make sure the team knows the patient's goals of care. Some tools that can assist in communication are written calendars, smartphone applications, and reminder phone calls.

▶ Screening and Prevention Guidelines

Two organizations that develop cancer screening guidelines are the US Preventive Services Task Force and the American Cancer Society. These guidelines are periodically revised based on systematic evidence reviews. Navigators need to keep up to date on the changing cancer screening recommendations and guidelines and be able to speak to patients regarding this important aspect of care. Early detection saves lives because cancer diagnosed at an earlier stage is easier to treat and has better outcomes.

Cancer-related checkups should include examination for cancers of the thyroid, testicles, ovaries, lymph nodes, oral cavity, and skin. Health counseling about tobacco, sun exposure, diet and nutrition, risk factors, sexual practices, and environmental and occupational exposures should be discussed at each checkup. Several organizations recommend a number of cancer screening guidelines. However, recommendations for screening for colon, breast, cervical, lung, and prostate cancer are very similar. The overall summary of screening guidelines for these five most common cancers is given in the following website: https://www.cancer.org/healthy/find-cancer-early /cancer-screening-guidelines/american-cancer-society-guidelines-for-the-early -detection-of-cancer.html. Every effort should be made to educate and reduce the barriers to screening. Healthcare providers need to take a more proactive approach. They should discuss these cancer screening guidelines with patients and recommend which test is most appropriate to increase patient awareness and promote long-term health. Patients must also take greater responsibility for their health to lower their risk for cancer.[8]

▶ Summary

Navigation is a dynamic and constantly changing field. The role of navigator was originally developed to help eliminate barriers to care and to promote timely diagnosis and treatment for cancer in underserved populations. Since its inception in the 1990s, the navigator role has grown across the disease trajectory and has helped to identify and eliminate communication, logistical, emotional/social, financial, and treatment-related barriers.

References

1. Freund KM, Battaglia TA, Calhoun E, et al. National Cancer Institute Patient Navigation Research Program: Methods, protocol, and measures. *Cancer*. 2008;113:3391–3399.
2. American College of Surgeons Commission on Cancer. Cancer Program Standards 2012: Version 1.2.1: Ensuring patient centered care. www.facs.org/quality%20programs/cancer/coc /standards. Accessed Sept 25, 2019.
3. Wright J, Williams R, Wilkinson JR. Development and importance of health needs assessment. *BMJ*. 1998;316:1310–1313.
4. Office of Disease Prevention and Health Promotion. US Department of Health and Human Services. Healthy people: Access to health services. www.healthypeople.gov/2020/topics -objectives/topic/Access-to-Health-Services. Accessed April 2019.
5. Blaseg KD, Daugherty P, Gamblin KA. *Oncology Nurse Navigation: Delivering Patient Centered Care Across the Continuum*. Pittsburgh, PA: Oncology Nursing Society, 2014.
6. McDougall JA, Ramsey SD, Shih YCT. Financial toxicity: A growing concern among cancer patients in the United States. www.ispor.org/news/articles/ISPORConnections_Vol20No2 _MarchApril2014.pdf. Accessed April 2019.
7. American Cancer Society. *Cancer Facts & Figures 2015*. Atlanta, GA: American Cancer Society, 2015. www.cancer.org/research/cancerfactsstatistics/cancerfactsfigures2015/index. Accessed April 2019.
8. American Cancer Society. American Cancer Society guidelines for the early detection of cancer. www.cancer.org/healthy/findcancerearly/cancerscreeningguidelines/american-cancer-society -guidelines-for-the-early-detection-of-cancer. Accessed April 2019.

Appendix C

AONN+ Evidence-Based Oncology Navigation Metrics Crosswalk with National Oncology Standards and Indicators*

Tricia Strusowski, MS, RN
Manager, Chartis Oncology Solutions

Danelle Johnston, MSN, RN, OCN, HON-ONN-CG
Chief Nursing Officer; Director of Strategic Planning and Initiatives

© Green Hill Healthcare. The Lynx Group

The first discussions about value-based metrics development for oncology navigation took place in November 2015 at the Academy of Oncology Nurse & Patient Navigators (AONN+) annual conference. Key stakeholders within the AONN+ membership identified an opportunity to develop quality outcome measures for navigation. It was recognized that the landscape of healthcare continued to evolve and focus on quality care measures and outcomes that impacts reimbursement. A proposal for the metrics development initiative was presented by the AONN+ Leadership Council and approved and funded by The Lynx Group in December 2015 (**FIGURE C-1**). In January 2016, the initiative was launched, led by Project Team Leader Tricia Strusowski, MS, RN, and Co-Project Team Leaders, Elaine Sein, BSN, RN, OCN, and Danelle Johnston, MSN, RN, OCN, HON-ONN-CG. A project team of content experts was organized (**FIGURE C-2**). This multidisciplinary team of 10 members was formed to create standardized navigation metrics focused on patient experience (PE), clinical outcomes (CO), and return on investment (ROI) utilizing the AONN+ knowledge domains as the framework for the metrics development (**TABLE C-1**).

The project team leaders held a Webex to roll out the project, timelines, and expectations of each team member and outlined the preparation required prior to retreat. Each member completed a literature review on the assigned domain for which they had validated expertise. The metrics team used measure development criteria ensuring feasibility, meaningfulness, and breadth of metric to attain reliability and validity. AONN+ held a 1-day retreat with the task force members to review

---

* This article was originally published in *Journal of Oncology Navigation & Survivorship* (2018; vol.9).

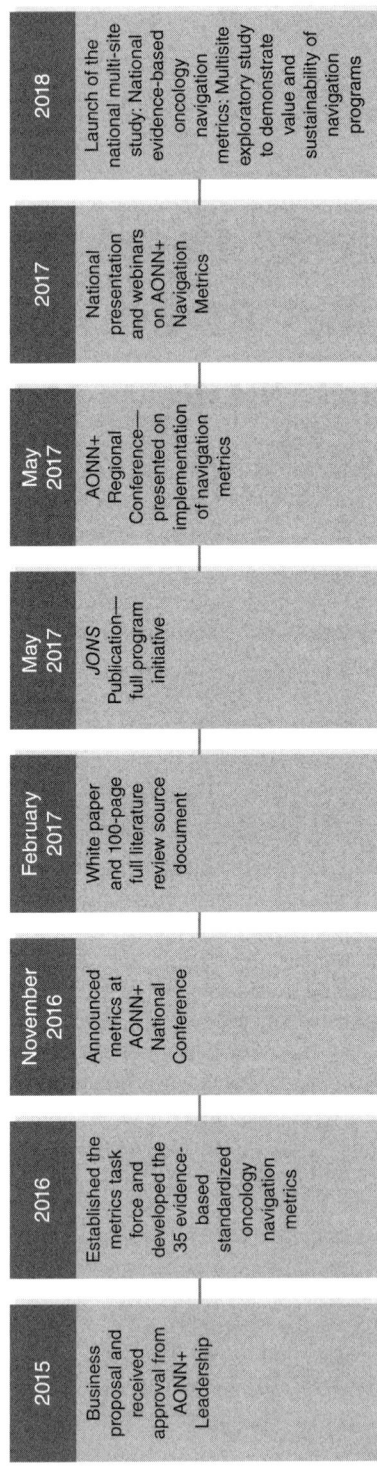

FIGURE C-1 Metrics Initiative Accomplishments to Date

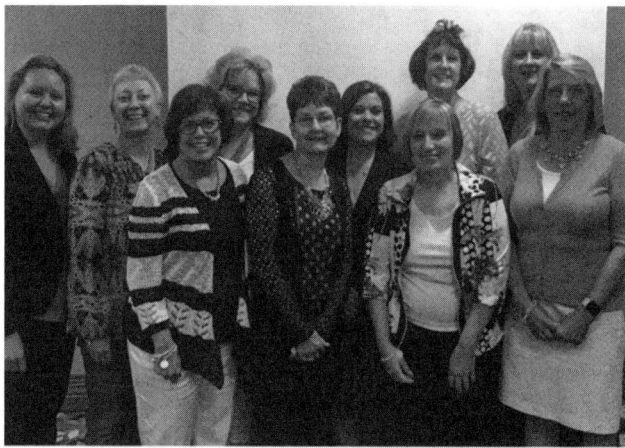

FIGURE C-2 AONN+ Standardized Metrics Team

From left to right: Vanessa Rodriguez, MSW, OPN-CG; Cheryl Bellomo, MSN, RN, OCN, ONN-CG; Barbara McHale, RN, BS, OCN, CBCN, ONN-CG; Tricia Strusowski, MS, RN; Elaine Sein, BSN, RN; Nicole Messier, BSN, RN, OCN, ONN-CG; Linda Bily, MA, CSA; Sharon Gentry, MSN, RN, CBCN, AOCN, ONN-CG; Danelle Johnston; MSN, RN, OCN, ONN-CG; and Elizabeth Brown, MSN, MHA, RN, OCN, NE-BC

© Green Hill Healthcare. Used with permission from Academy of Oncology Nurse & Patient Navigators.

metrics, literature support, and benchmarks for each domain and [to] finalize a set of standard metrics. Using a Likert scale, the team ranked metrics to determine which met rigorous review and were acknowledged as being of high validity that all navigation programs can utilize.

The creation of these standardized national metrics to measure programmatic success is vital to coordinating high-quality, team-based care and demonstrating the sustainability of navigation programs. It is imperative that oncology nurse and patient navigators understand that active participation in data collection, analytics, and reporting outcomes are not added responsibilities but are already a part of the professional role. The implications for navigation practices using quality navigation measures are that they are transformative, evaluate professional practice and care delivery, define oncology navigation practice and outcomes, and are necessary for sustainability of navigation.[1-3]

The outcome of this initial work was the publication of 35 standardized, evidence-based, oncology navigation metrics. To view the measures in their entirety, please reference the *AONN+ Standardized Metrics Source Document* (www .aonnonline.org/metrics-source-document). To read the full project implementation, please access the May 2017 issue of the *Journal of Oncology Navigation & Survivorship* (www.jons-online.com/issue-archive/2017-issues/may-2017-vol-8-no-5).

AONN+ recognizes that navigation programs are developing at different rates within diverse structural organizations and settings that will determine which standardized metrics will be essential to measure outcomes for their specific navigation program. As disease-specific certification evolves, additional evidence-based disease-specific metrics will need to be developed to dovetail into the standardized navigation metrics.

The US healthcare system is the costliest in the world. It is projected that by 2026, 20% of the gross national product will be spent on healthcare.[4] In light of the growing aging populations and chronic health conditions, there is a global challenge to provide cost-effective quality healthcare. The landscape of healthcare has shifted, driven by the Triple Aim to reduce cost per capita in healthcare, improve the PE of care, and advance health outcomes. It is essential for outcomes to be driven by standardized evidence-based metrics that can effectively be measured with the

TABLE C-1 AONN+ Knowledge Domains

- Community Outreach and Prevention
- Coordination of Care/Care Transitions
- Patient Advocacy/Patient Empowerment
- Psychosocial Support Services/Assessment
- Survivorship/End of Life
- Professional Roles and Responsibilities
- Operations Management/Organizational
- Development/Healthcare Economics
- Research/Quality/Performance Improvement

application of data analytics and implementation of performance improvement initiatives. National standards with value-based care are now propelling cancer programs to be accountable and measure both quality of care delivery and cost.

Quality care is defined by the Institute of Medicine (IOM) as the "[d]egree in which health services [knowledge] for individuals and populations increase the likelihood of desired health outcomes and are consistent with current professional knowledge [research evidence]."[5]

The IOM has identified gaps in cancer quality care—gaps in existing measures; challenges with measure development; lack of consumer engagement in measure development and reporting; and data to support meaningful, timely, actionable performance measures.[6] IOM stated, "To ensure the rapid translation of research into practice, a mechanism is needed to quickly identify the results of research with quality-of-care implications and ensure that it is applied in monitoring quality."[7] Providers, including healthcare systems, health plans, physicians, program administrators, and navigators must be held accountable for demonstrating that they provide and improve quality of care through quality measures. A core set of indicators need[s] to be collected to measure and monitor quality of care that span the continuum of cancer care.[7]

Jojola and colleagues completed a systematic review of literature evaluating 15 peer-reviewed articles assessing patient navigation efficacy for cancer patients undergoing treatment. The review identified the need for heterogeneity[,] a consistent way in which data are reported to allow for better assessments in research. The authors also acknowledge the need for metrics to evaluate the outcomes of patient navigation throughout the cancer care trajectory to assess its effectiveness. Jojola [et al. state], "Improving standardization of patient navigation metrics would allow clinicians, policy makers, patients, and other researchers to better measure the impact of patient navigation across the continuum of cancer care."[8] It is imperative for navigation to continue to build a strong sustainable business case through the collection, measurement, and reporting of the 35 newly established standardized metrics. Harnessing the power of this information to create best practices will elevate navigation and garner industry support for advancing patient-centered care delivery.

The AONN+ standardized oncology navigation metrics focus on PE, CO, and ROI that align with national oncology standards and indicators. These national standards and indicators are defined by the Commission on Cancer (CoC) National Accreditation Program, the National Accreditation Program for Breast Centers

(NAPBC), the Oncology Care Model (OCM), the Quality Oncology Practice Initiative (QOPI), and the Medicare Access and CHIP Reauthorization Act (MACRA). AONN+ developed a crosswalk taking the 35 standardized metrics and identifying how these measures align with the national standards and indicators. A complete list of those national standards that support AONN+ Metrics follow this article (**TABLES C-2 TO C-9**). Additional background data are provided to define the national standards and indicators and how these dovetail with AONN+ metrics. Administrators, providers, and navigators need to be harmonizing to see how the national measures and indicators align and work in metric synergy. Through the cancer program goals, they can identify national standards and indicators that cross the cancer care trajectory, creating strong metrics that do not cause metric silos.

▶ Oncology National Standards and Measures

Commission on Cancer

Over the past 80 years, the CoC has been engaged in the definition and recognition of quality cancer care. The emphasis is on improving overall survival and quality of life for cancer patients that addresses standard-setting to advance cancer prevention, research, education, and monitoring of quality care delivery.[9] The CoC initiatives are currently led by 56 representatives from professional organizations. The CoC has established patient-centered standards and quality measures to support delivery of multidisciplinary delivery of high-quality cancer care. The National Cancer Database (NCDBC) is utilized by the CoC to collect, analyze, and report cancer program data.[10] Both the Cancer Program Practice Profile Reports and the Rapid Quality Reporting System are used to facilitate real-time reporting, auditing, and updating of data.

Currently, there are approximately 1,500 CoC national accredited programs across the United States, including Puerto Rico. The accreditation focuses programs to improve their quality of care delivery through the implementation of national standards and measures. The focus on cancer care delivery starts at prevention and moves through the cancer care continuum into survivorship and end of life. There are 5 areas of focus: (1) Program Management, (2) Clinical Services, (3) Continuum of Care Services, (4) Patient Outcomes, and (5) Data Quality, with a total of 34 standards that are evaluated within the accreditation process. The CoC Cancer Program Standards: Ensuring Patient-Centered Care can be accessed on the CoC website at https://www.facs.org/quality-programs/cancer/ncdb.[11]

National Accreditation Program for Breast Center

The NAPBC is a consortium of national professional organizations committed to the improvement of quality care and monitoring outcomes (**TABLE C-10**). The three pillars focus on standard-setting, scientific validation, and patient and professional education. The six domains focus on (1) Center Leadership, (2) Clinical Services, (3) Research, (4) Community Outreach, (5) Professional Outreach, and (6) Quality Improvement.[12] A total of 26 quality standards are required for programs to demonstrate successful achievement.

TABLE C-2 NAPBC-Accredited Centers Demonstrate the Following Services

- A multidisciplinary team approach to coordinate the best care and treatment options available
- Access to breast-specific information, education, and support
- Breast center data collection on quality indicators for subspecialties involved in breast cancer diagnosis and treatment
- Ongoing monitoring and improvement of care
- Information about participation in clinical trials and new treatment options

National Accreditation Program for Breast Centers. *Standards Manual.* 2018 Edition. https://accreditation.facs.org /accreditationdocuments/NAPBC/Portal%20Resources/2018NAPBCStandardsManual.pdf. Accessed May 1, 2018.

Oncology Care Model

The Centers for Medicare & Medicaid Services (CMS) have designed new episode-based payment and care delivery models with the outcome to drive improvement in overall health outcomes and high-quality care and provide highly coordinated care at the same or lower cost for oncology patients (**FIGURE C-3**). This 5-year model was launched July 1, 2016, and will end June 30, 2021, and will be evaluating episodes of care that include chemotherapy at 6-month intervals. Participating in the OCM are 184 practices and 13 payers.[13] The goal is to drive practice transformation utilizing aligned financial incentives that include performance-based incentives, which increase value of services while decreasing unnecessary utilization of services.

The model was designed utilizing the National Quality Strategy, which focused on four quality measures: (1) Communication and care coordination, (2) Person- and caregiver-centered experience, (3) Clinical quality of care outcomes, and (4) Patient safety. The four measures align with the standardized metrics developed by AONN+ focused on PE, CO, and ROI. See **TABLE C-11** for the 12 quality measures that impact performance-based payment and are measured and reported at quarterly intervals to drive continuous quality improvement and identify best practices.[14]

Quality Oncology Practice Initiative

QOPI was initiated in 2010 to enhance the services provided to the oncology patients by raising the quality of care provided and monitored in the oncology medical and hematology oncology physicians' offices.[15] QOPI surveys the individual practices in over 100 different measures. The metrics follow national guidelines and incorporate services that provide exceptional care for the cancer patient.

QOPI has standardized best practices in regard to PE, CO, and ROI. These metrics assist medical oncologists and their staff with facilitating critical conversations with their patients, such as patients' goals of care and treatment wishes, and fruitful open discussions about clinical treatment options and outcomes. These conversations are extremely valuable from the patients' perspective. The IOM noted in its report, *Delivering High-Quality Cancer Care: Charting a New Course for a System in Crisis,*[16] that the patients want involvement. The number 1 response from patients when asked "What do you want from your provider?" was "I want my provider to

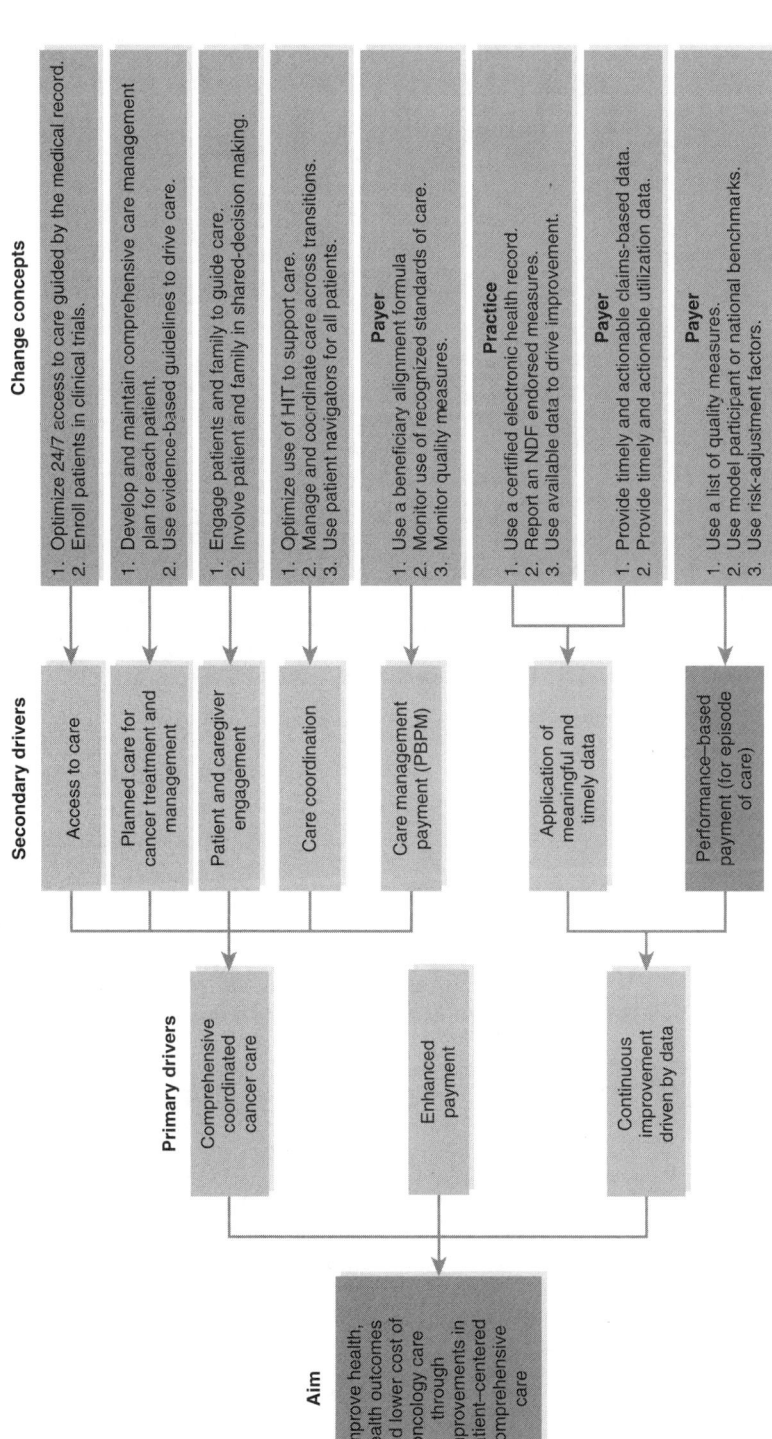

FIGURE C-3 Oncology Care Model Driver Diagram

Centers for Medicare & Medicaid Services. Oncology Care Model. https://innovation.cms.gov/Files/x/ocmfa.pdf. Accessed May 4, 2018.

TABLE C-3 Measures to Be Used in OCM Performance Multiplier

Measure Name	OCM Measure Number	Measure Source
Communication and Care Coordination		
Risk-adjusted proportion of patients with all-cause hospital admissions within the 6-month episode	OCM-1	Claims
Risk-adjusted proportion of patients with all-cause emergency department visits or observation stays that did not result in a hospital admission within the 6-month episode	OCM-2	Claims
Proportion of patients who died who were admitted to hospice for 3 days or more	OCM-3	Claims
Person- and caregiver-centered experience and outcomes		
Pain assessment and management composite*	OCM-4	Registry (practice-reported)
Preventive care and screening: screening for depression and follow-up plan (CMS 2v6.3, National Quality forum (NQF) 0418)	OCM-5	Registry (practice-reported)
Patient-reported experience of care	OCM-6	Survey
Clinical quality of care outcomes		
Prostate cancer: adjuvant hormonal therapy for high- or very high-risk prostate cancer (PQRS 104, NQF 0390)[†]	OCM-7	Registry (practice-reported)
Adjuvant chemotherapy is recommended or administered within 4 months (120 days) of diagnosis to patients under the age of 80 with the American Joint Committee on Cancer Staging (AJCC) III (lymph node–positive) colon cancer (NQF 0223)	OCM-8	Registry (practice-reported)
Combination chemotherapy is recommended or administered within 4 months (120 days) of diagnosis for women under 70 with AJCC T1cN0M0, or state IB-III hormone receptor–negative breast cancer (NQF 0559)	OCM-9	Registry (practice-reported)

Clinical quality of care outcomes		
Trastuzumab administered to patients with AJCC stage I (T1c)-III and human epidermal growth factor receptor 2 (HER2) positive breast cancer who receive adjuvant chemotherapy (NQF 1858)	OCM-10	Registry (practice-reported)
Breast Cancer: hormonal therapy for stage I (T1b)-IIIC estrogen receptor/progesterone Receptor (ER/PR) Positive breast cancer (CMS 140v5.0, NQF 0387)	OCM-11	Registry (practice-reported)
Patient safety		
Documentation of current medications in the medical record (CMS 68v6.1, NQF 0419)	OCMM-12	Registry (practice-reported)

* The composite measure, OCM-4, is comprised of 2 measures: OCM-4a, Oncology: Medical and Radiation—Pain Intensity Quantified (PQRS 143, NQF 0384), and OCM-4b, Oncology: Medical and Radiation—Plan of Care for Pain (PQRS 144, NQF 0383).
† OCM-7 was retired effective with the March 2018 reporting period.
Oncology Care Model. OCM Performance-Based Payment Methodology. Version 2.1. December 27, 2017. https://innovation.cms.gov/initiatives/Oncology-Care. Accessed May 2, 2016.

listen to me" (**FIGURE C-4**). Patients want more than ever to have their voices heard, and they want the best clinical care and their life goals discussed. Having these conversations earlier in the continuum provides superb clinical care and supports patient- and family-centered care. Achieving excellence in cancer care is a goal of QOPI, keeping the patient and family involved with discussions and providing the highest level of quality across the entire continuum of care. QOPI certification demonstrates the physician commitment to quality oncology care to the patient and their family in regard to national standards. When reviewing the goals from the IOM, the first and second goals are directly related to the patient (**TABLE C-12**).[16]

QOPI is a voluntary program to help medical oncology and hematology/oncology practices evaluate the quality of the care they provide to patients. Data are collected and compared to more than 100 quality measures (aspects of care based on published care recommendations and expert opinion). To achieve QOPI certification, a practice must have participated in QOPI and met or exceeded a benchmark score on measures that compared the quality of its care against national standards. A practice then undergoes an on-site review and peer review by a select team of oncology professionals, such as physicians and nurses, at least once every 3 years. Certification is awarded when a practice meets the QOPI Certification Program standards.[15]

Medicare Access and CHIP Reauthorization Act

MACRA is legislation signed into law April 16, 2015. MACRA created the Quality Payment Program (QPP) that repeals the Sustainable Growth Rate formula, changes the way Medicare rewards clinicians for value over volume, streamlines multiple quality

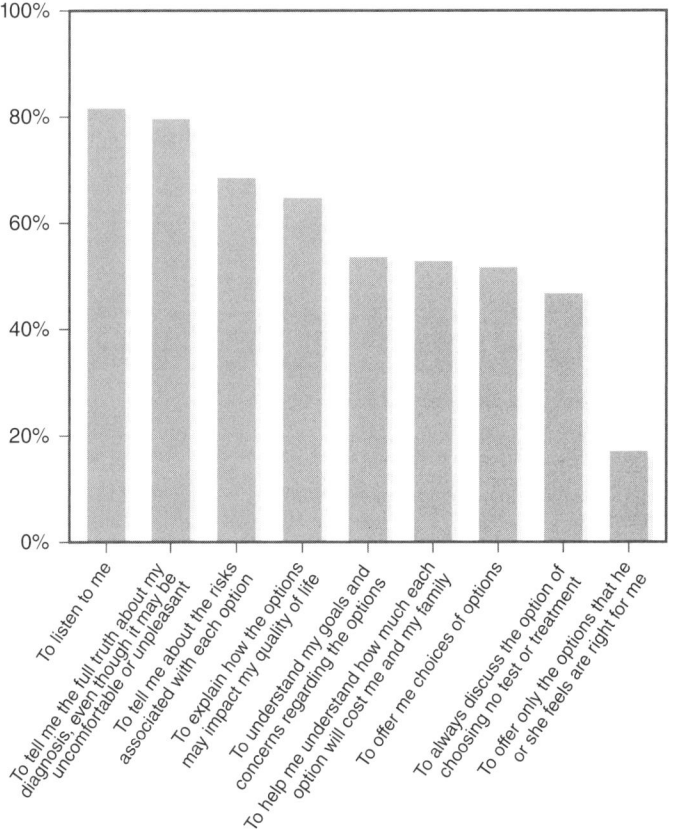

People want involvement in evidence and decisions
Bars show the percent of people surveyed who <u>strongly agree</u>
with the statement:"I want my provider..."

FIGURE C-4 Patients Want Involvement

TABLE C-4 Goals of the Recommendations from the IOM

1. Provide clinical and cost information to patients.
2. End-of-life care consistent with patients' values.
3. Coordinated, team-based cancer care.
4. Core competencies for the workforce.
5. Expand breadth of cancer research data.
6. Expand depth of cancer research data.
7. Develop a learning healthcare information technology (IT) system for cancer.
8. A national quality reporting program for cancer care.
9. Reduce disparities in access to cancer care.
10. Improve the affordability of cancer care.

Modified from Institute of Medicine. *Delivering High-Quality Cancer Care: Charting a New Course for a System in Crisis*. Washington, DC: The National Academies Press, 2013.

programs under the new Merit-based Incentive Payments System (MIPS), and gives bonus payments for participation in eligible Alternative Payment Models (APMs).[17]

The MACRA QPP includes quality improvement activities, advancing care information, and cost.[18]

The landmark passage of MACRA marked one of the most significant changes to Medicare legislation the healthcare industry has seen.

Clinicians can adopt two reporting tracks when participating in MACRA—MIPS and APMs.[19]

MIPS indicators are not entirely foreign to providers; they are used to measures included in meaningful use and the Physician Quality Reporting System.

APMs is a payment approach that gives added incentive payments to provide high-quality and cost-efficient care. APMs can apply to a specific clinical condition, a care episode, or a population.[19]

A review of the MIPS/APMs indicators shows that they cross all AONN+ domains. For example, they address clinical coordination of care, operations management, community screening, psychosocial screening, and survivorship, also known as patient self-management. MIPS/APMs metrics also are very similar to the QOPI indicators with regard to PE, CO, and ROI.

The foundation of the MIPS and APMs programs is the delivery of high-quality patient care. Using a variety of tools, physicians report data to CMS, receive valuable feedback about their practice, and are eligible for payment adjustments.

How does the QPP benefit clinicians and patients? The clinicians benefit from streamlined reporting, standardized measures (evidence-based), and eliminated duplicative reporting, which allow[s] them to spend more time with patients, promote industry alignment through multipayer models, and incentivize care that focuses on improved quality outcomes. The patients benefit by increased access to better care, enhanced coordination through a patient-centered approach, and improved results.[19]

The payment model will be based on quality performance during a 90-day episode of care. The QPP incentivizes providers to participate, utilizing their indicators of choice and ensuring high-quality care through incentive payments from Medicare.

The QPP Strategic Goals[19]

- Improve beneficiary outcomes
- Increase adoption of advanced APMs
- Improve data and information sharing
- Enhance clinician experience
- Maximize participation
- Ensure operational excellence in program implementation

▶ Summary

Whereas oncology navigation programs have been in existence for decades, there is an evident gap in the literature around metrics. This gap has resulted in the lack of solid benchmarks and limited research in navigation. Navigation services are not reimbursable to date, and administrators need to take the lead with their navigation programs to create metrics that support value-based cancer care.[20] Value-based cancer care metrics for an oncology program need to include national oncology guidelines such as CoC, NAPBC, oncology national quality standards such as QOPI, and payment modules such as OCM, and MIPS/APMs that support PE, CO, and ROI.

In today's healthcare landscape, it is essential for cancer programs to harmonize their performance improvement initiatives or create "metric synergy." Presently, providers, administrators, clinical trials departments, and navigation programs are all collecting metrics in silos. There is strength and sustainability in synergy. As oncology resources become more limited and oncology physicians fewer in number, it will be essential that each provider and midlevel and professional staff member work to the top of their licensure in their state. The creation of standing order sets, pathways, and guidelines will support value-based cancer care metrics and be essential ingredients to oncology programs. Processes and role delineation will ensure [that] the team is functioning to its highest level with the patient and their family in the center, resulting in clinical excellence, the ultimate goal.

When collecting metrics, it is essential that each team member understands the program goals and performance improvement metrics to achieve these goals. Each team member is a vital link to enhancing the cancer program; thus all have a specific role when it comes to incorporating metrics into the day-to-day operations of the cancer program. Providers, administrators, and oncology program department heads need to discuss the goals of their cancer program and select metrics that support these goals. The goals then need to be shared with every staff member in the cancer program. Each staff member needs to be fully aware of the cancer program metrics, the definition, the desired outcome, and the benefits of meeting and exceeding the metrics. The ultimate goal for the program is to provide the highest level of engaged patient- and family-centered care with CO resulting in a high ROI.

References

1. Barnsteiner J, Reeder VC, Palma WH, et al. Promoting evidence-based practice and translational research. *Nurs Adm Q.* 2010;34:217–225.
2. Crane-Okada R. Evaluation and outcome measure in patient navigation. *Semin Oncol Nurs.* 2013;29:128–140.
3. Guadagnolo B, Dohan D, Raich P. Metrics for evaluating patient navigation during cancer diagnosis and treatment: Crafting a policy-relevant research agenda for patient navigation in cancer care. *Cancer.* 2011;117(15 suppl):3565–3574.
4. Centers for Medicare & Medicaid Services. NHE Fact Sheet. www.cms.gov/research-statistics-data-and-systems/statistics-trends-and-reports/nationalhealthexpenddata/nhe-fact-sheet .html. Accessed May 1, 2018.
5. Institute of Medicine. *Crossing the Quality Chasm: A New Health System for the 21st Century.* Washington, DC: National Academies Press, 2001.
6. Institute of Medicine. *The Future of Nursing: Leading the Change Advancing the Health.* Washington, DC: National Academies Press, 2010.
7. Institute of Medicine. *Ensuring Quality Cancer Care.* Washington, DC: National Academies Press, 1999.
8. Jojola CE, Cheng H, Wong LJ, et al. Efficacy of patient navigation in cancer treatment: A systematic review. *J Oncol Navig Surviv.* 2017;8:106–115.
9. Commission on Cancer. www.facs.org/quality-programs/cancer/coc. Accessed May 1, 2018.
10. Commission on Cancer. Cancer Program Standards: Ensuring Patient-Centered Care. www .facs.org/~/media/files/quality%20programs/cancer/coc/2016%20coc%20standards%20 manual_interactive%20pdf.ashx. 2016. Accessed May 1, 2018.
11. Commission on Cancer. Cancer Program Standards: Ensuring Patient-Centered Care. https:// www.facs.org/quality-programs/cancer/. Accessed May 2016.

12. National Accreditation Program for Breast Centers. *Standards Manual*. 2018 Edition. https:// accreditation.facs.org/accreditationdocuments/NAPBC/Portal%20Resources/2018NAPBC-StandardsManual.pdf. Accessed May 1, 2018.
13. Centers for Medicare & Medicaid Services. Oncology Care Model. https://innovation.cms.gov /initiatives/Oncology-Care. Accessed May 1, 2018.
14. Oncology Care Model. OCM Performance-Based Payment Methodology. Version 2.1. December 27, 2017. https://innovation.cms.gov/initiatives/Oncology-Care. Accessed May 2, 2016.
15. Cancer.net.www.cancer.net/about-us/about-asco/about-qopi%C2%AE-certification-program. Accessed April 30, 2018.
16. Institute of Medicine. *Delivering High-Quality Cancer Care: Charting a New Course for a System in Crisis*. Washington, DC: The National Academies Press, 2013. www.cms.gov. Accessed April 30, 2018.
17. The Health Management Academy and PerfectServe. Making Sense of MACRA. www.perfect-serve.com/macra-webinar. March 2017. Accessed April 1, 2016.
18. Centers for Medicare & Medicaid Services. The Merit-based Incentive Payment System: MIPS Scoring Methodology Overview. March 2017. www.cms.gov/Medicare/Quality-Initia-tives-Patient-Assessment-Instruments/Value-Based-Programs/MACRA-MIPS-and-APMs/ MIPS-Scoring-Methodology-slide-deck.pdf. Accessed April 1, 2016.
19. Strusowski T. Creating value in cancer care through standardized metrics and partnerships. *J Clin Pathways*. 2018;4(3):42–47.

TABLE C-5 National Standards in Support of AONN+ Metrics within Community Outreach, Prevention Domain

AONN+ METRIC: Cancer screening follow-up to diagnostic workup—number of navigated patients per quarter with abnormal screening referred for follow-up diagnostic workup.* (PE, CO, ROI)	
Association	**Standard**
CoC	Standard 1.8: Each calendar year, the Community Outreach Co-ordinator, under the direction of the cancer committee, monitors the effectiveness of prevention, screening, and outreach activities
	Standard 4.2: Each calendar year, the cancer committee organizes and offers at least 1 cancer screening program that is designed to decrease the number of patients with late-stage disease and is targeted to meet the screening needs of the community. Each screening program is consistent with evidence-based national guidelines and interventions and must have a formal process developed to follow up on all positive findings
NAPBC	Standard 4.1: Education, Prevention and Early Detection Programs
	Each year, 2 or more breast cancer education, prevention, and/or early detection programs are provided on site or coordinated with other facilities or local agencies targeted to the community, and *follow-up is provided* to patient with positive findings

(continues)

TABLE C-5 National Standards in Support of AONN+ Metrics within Community Outreach, Prevention Domain   *(continued)*

AONN+ METRIC: Cancer screening follow-up to diagnostic workup—number of navigated patients per quarter with abnormal screening referred for follow-up diagnostic workup.* (PE, CO, ROI)

Association	Standard
Quality Payment Program (QPP) The Merit-based Incentive Payment System (MIPS) Advanced Alternative Payment Models (Advanced APMs)	Breast cancer screening. Measure ID: 112
	Colorectal cancer screening. Measure ID: 113
	Preventive care and screening: tobacco use: screening and cessation intervention. Measure ID: 226
	Smoking abstinence. Measure ID: Anesthesia Quality Institute (AQI) 16
	Tobacco use: screening and cessation intervention. Measure ID: PPRNET 23
	Cervical cancer screening. Measure ID: 309
	Screening colonoscopy adenoma detection rate. Measure ID: 343
	Cervical cancer screening measure. ID: PPRNET 16
	Breast cancer screening. Measure ID: PPRNET 17
	Colorectal cancer screening measure ID: PPRNET 18
	Optimizing patient exposure to ionizing radiation: appropriateness: follow-up CT imaging for incidentally detected pulmonary nodules according to recommended guidelines. Measure ID: 364
	Screening for hepatocellular carcinoma (HCC) in patients with hepatitis C cirrhosis. Measure ID: 401

AONN+ METRIC: Cancer screening—number of participants at cancer screening event and/or percentage increase of cancer screening. (PE, CO)

Association	Standard*
CoC	Report name of program, type of cancer, date of program screening, national guidelines followed, outline process for follow-up on positive findings, results and summary of effectiveness
	Can evaluate number of individuals screened compared to prior year and coordinate with other departments providing screenings (mobile mammography or breast health center)
	Standard 4.1: Cancer prevention programs
	Standard 4.2: Cancer screening program: each calendar year, the cancer committee organizes and offers at least 1 cancer screening

AONN+ METRIC: Cancer screening—number of participants at cancer screening event and/or percentage increase of cancer screening. (PE, CO)	
Association	**Standard***
NAPBC	Type of program, location, target audience, coordinated with number of participants
	Describe the process used to follow up with patients found to have positive findings as a result of participation in early detection programs
	Standard 4.1: Education, prevention and early detection

* Cancer screening definition: Screening tests can help find cancer at an early stage before symptoms will appear. When abnormal tissue or cancer is found early, it may be easier to treat or cure. By the time symptoms appear, the cancer may have grown and spread. This can make cancer more difficult to treat or cure.

TABLE C-6 National Standards in Support of AONN+ Metrics within Care Coordination/Care Transitions Domain

AONN+ METRIC: Percentage of navigated patients who adhere to institutional treatment pathways per quarter. (CO, ROI)	
Association	**Standard**
CoC	Standards 4.4 and 4.5
	Each calendar year, the expected Estimated Performance Rate is met for each
	Accountability and quality improvement measures as defined by the CoC
	CoC programs are required to submit data to the Rapid Quality Reporting System (RQRS) (breast and colorectal) real-time monitoring of treatment compliance monthly or quarterly
NAPBC	Annual breast program leadership (BPL) monitored
	Standard 2.3: Breast conservation stages 0, I, II
	Standard 2.4: Sentinel lymph node biopsy (Bx) rate
	Standard 2.8: Needle biopsy rate
	Standard 2.18: Reconstructive surgery referral rate
QOPI	13a1: Chemotherapy administered to patients with metastatic solid tumor with performance status of 3, 4, or undocumented. (lower score is better) (top 5 measure) (defect-free measure 13a1a, 13a1b)
	13a1a: Chemotherapy administered to patients with metastatic solid tumor with performance status of 3 or 4 (lower score is better) (top 5 measure)
	13a1b: Chemotherapy administered to patients with metastatic solid tumor with performance status undocumented (lower score is better) (top 5 measure)

(continues)

TABLE C-6 National Standards in Support of AONN+ Metrics within Care Coordination/Care Transitions Domain   *(continued)*

AONN+ METRIC: Percentage of navigated patients who adhere to institutional treatment pathways per quarter. (CO, ROI)

Association	Standard
	13oc4: Documented plan for oral chemotherapy (defect-free measure, 13oc4a–13oc4d) (test measure)
	13oc4a: Documented plan for oral chemotherapy: dose
	13oc4b: Documented plan for oral chemotherapy: administration schedule (start day, days of treatment/rest and planned duration)
	13oc4c: Documented plan for oral chemotherapy: provided to patient/caregiver prior to start of therapy and practitioner(s) providing continuing care within 3 months of starting therapy (test measure)
	13oc4d: Documented plan for oral chemotherapy: indications
	26: Serotonin antagonist prescribed or administered with moderate/high emetic risk chemotherapy
	27: Corticosteroids and serotonin antagonist prescribed or administered with moderate/high emetic risk chemotherapy*
	28: Neurokinin-1 receptor (NK1) receptor antagonist and olanzapine prescribed or administered with high emetic risk chemotherapy
	Symptom/Toxicity 28a NK1 receptor antagonist (aprepitant/fosaprepitant/netupitant) and olanzapine administered for low or moderate emetic risk cycle 1 chemotherapy (lower score is better) (top 5 test measure)
	29: Antiemetics prescribed or administered appropriately with moderate/moderate-/high emetic risk chemotherapy (defect-free measure 27 and 28)
	52: Combination chemotherapy recommended within 4 months of diagnosis for women under the age of 70 with AJCC stage IA (T1c) and IB-III ER/PR-negative breast cancer. NQF endorsed #0559 (adapted)
	52a: Complete staging for women with invasive breast cancer (cancer stage, HER2neu, and estrogen/progesterone (ER/PR) status)
	53: Combination chemotherapy received within 4 months of diagnosis by women under the age of 70 with AJCC stage IA (T1c) and IB-III ER/PR-negative breast cancer.* NQF endorsed #0559 (adapted)
	54: Test for HER2neu overexpression or gene amplification.* NQF endorsed #1878 (adapted)
	Breast 55: Trastuzumab recommended for patients with AJCC stage I (T1c) to III HER2neu–positive breast cancer. NQF endorsed #1858 (adapted)

AONN+ METRIC: Percentage of navigated patients who adhere to institutional treatment pathways per quarter. (CO, ROI)	
Association	**Standard**
	56: Trastuzumab received when Her-2/neu is negative or undocumented (lower score is better). NQF endorsed #1857 (adapted)
	Breast 56a: Trastuzumab not received when Her-2/neu is negative or undocumented (inverse of 56).* NQF endorsed #1857 (adapted)
	57: Trastuzumab received by patients with AJCC IA (T1c) and IB-III Her-2/neu–positive breast cancer.* NQF endorsed #1858 (adapted)
	Breast 58: Tamoxifen or AI recommended within 1 year of diagnosis for patients with AJCC stage IA (T1c) and IB-III ER- or PR-positive breast cancer. NQF endorsed #0220/#0387 (adapted)
	59: Tamoxifen or AI received within 1 year of diagnosis by patients with AJCC stage IA(T1c) and IB-III ER- or PR-positive breast cancer.* NQF endorsed #0220/#0387 (adapted)
	Breast 60: Tamoxifen or AI received when ER/PR status is negative or undocumented (lower score is better)
	61: Bone-modifying agents (IV bisphosphonates or denosumab)
	62: Renal function assessed prior to the first administration of IV bisphosphonates or denosumab
	62a1: PET, Cat Scan (CT), or radionuclide bone scan ordered by practice within 60 days after diagnosis to stage I, IIA, or IIB breast cancer (lower score is better) (top 5 measure)
	62a2: PET, CT, or radionuclide bone scan ordered outside of practice within 60 days after diagnosis to stage I, IIA, or IIB breast cancer (lower score is better) (top 5 measure)
	62b1: PET, CT, or radionuclide bone scan ordered by practice between day 61 and day 365 after diagnosis of breast cancer in patients who received treatment with curative intent (lower score is better) (top 5 measure)
	62b2: PET, CT, or radionuclide bone scan ordered outside of practice between day 61 and day 365 after diagnosis of breast cancer in patients who received treatment with curative intent (lower score is better) (top 5 measure)
	62c1: Serum tumor marker surveillance ordered by practice between 30 days and 365 days after diagnosis of breast cancer in patients who received treatment with curative intent for breast cancer (lower score is better) (top 5 measure)
	62c2: Serum tumor marker surveillance ordered outside of practice between 30 days and 365 days after diagnosis of breast cancer in patients who received treatment with curative intent for breast cancer (lower score is better) (top 5 measure)
	62d: Granulocyte colony-stimulating factor (GCSF) administered to patients who received chemotherapy for metastatic breast cancer (lower score is better) (top 5 measure)

(continues)

TABLE C-6 National Standards in Support of AONN+ Metrics within Care Coordination/Care Transitions Domain *(continued)*

AONN+ METRIC: Percentage of navigated patients who adhere to institutional treatment pathways per quarter. (CO, ROI)

Association	Standard
	66: CEA within 4 months of curative resection for colorectal cancer*
	67: Adjuvant chemotherapy recommended within 4 months of diagnosis for patients with AJCC stage III colon cancer. NQF endorsed #0223/#0385 (adapted)
	Colorectal 68: Adjuvant chemotherapy received within 4 months of diagnosis by patients with AJCC stage III colon cancer.* NQF endorsed #0223/#0385 (adapted)
	70: 12 or more lymph nodes examined for resected colon cancer. NQF endorsed #0225 (adapted)
	Colorectal 71: Adjuvant chemotherapy recommended within 9 months of diagnosis by patients with AJCC stage II or III rectal cancer
	73: Colonoscopy before or within 6 months of curative colorectal resection or completion of primary adjuvant chemotherapy.* NQF endorsed #1859 (adapted)
	Colorectal 74: RAS (KRAS and NRAS) testing for patients with metastatic colorectal cancer who received anti-EGFR MoAb therapy.* NQF endorsed #1860 (adapted)
	75: Anti-EGFR MoAb therapy received by patients with *KRAS* and *NRAS* mutation (lower score is better) (top 5 measure). NQF endorsed #1860 (adapted)
	75a: Anti-EGFR MoAb therapy not received by patients with *KRAS* and *NRAS* mutation (inverse of 75)*
	75b: GCSF administered to patients who received chemotherapy for metastatic colon cancer (lower score is better) (top 5 measure)
	76: Percentage of colon cancer patients with PET or PET-CT ordered by practice after the completion of treatment with curative intent for colon cancer (lower score is better) (top 5 measure)
	77msi: Proportion of patients with a diagnosis of colorectal cancer who had microsatellite instability (MSI) status determined by MSI analysis or immunohistochemistry by mismatched repair proteins
	78: Proportion of patients with a diagnosis of nonmetastatic rectal cancer who received a transrectal ultrasound or pelvic MRI to determine the stage of disease prior to initial therapy or surgery (test measure)
	77: Obinutuzumab, ofatumumab, or rituximab administered when CD antigen expression is negative or undocumented (lower score is better)

AONN + METRIC: Percentage of navigated patients who adhere to institutional treatment pathways per quarter. (CO, ROI)	
Association	**Standard**
	77a: Obinutuzumab, ofatumumab, or rituximab not administered when CD antigen expression is negative or undocumented (inverse of 77)
	78a: Hepatitis B virus infection test (HBsAg) and hepatitis B core antibody (anti-HBc) test within 3 months prior to initiation of obinutuzumab, ofatumumab, or rituximab for patients with non-Hodgkins lymphoma (NHL)
	79: Adjuvant chemotherapy recommended for patients with AJCC stage II or IIIA non-small-cell lung carcinoma (NSCLC)
	80n: Percentage of patients with PET or PET-CT ordered by practice between 3 and 12 months after completion of treatment with curative intent for diffuse large B-cell lymphoma (lower score is better) (top 5 measure)
	80: Adjuvant chemotherapy received by patients with AJCC stage II or IIIA NSCLC
	81: Adjuvant cisplatin-based chemotherapy received within 60 days after curative resection by patients with AJCC stage II or IIIA NSCLC*
	82: Adjuvant chemotherapy recommended for patients with AJCC stage IA NSCLC (lower score is better)
	83: Adjuvant radiation therapy recommended for patients with AJCC stage IB or II NSCLC (lower score is better)
	NSCLC 84: Performance status documented for patients with initial AJCC stage IV or distant metastatic NSCLC*
	85: Platinum doublet first-line chemotherapy or EGFR-TKI (or other targeted therapy with documented DNA mutation) received by patients with initial AJCC stage IV or distant metastatic NSCLC with performance status of 0-1 without prior history of chemotherapy*
	86a: Bevacizumab received by patients with initial AJCC stage IV or distant metastatic NSCLC with squamous histology (lower score is better)
	88: Patients with stage IV NSCLC with adenocarcinoma histology with an activating *EGFR* mutation or anaplastic lymphoma kinase (*ALK*) gene rearrangement who received first-line epidermal growth factor receptor (EGFR) tyrosine kinase inhibitor or other targeted therapy*
	89: Patients with stage IV NSCLC with *EGFR* mutation status unknown or without an activating *EGFR* mutation or *ALK* gene rearrangement who received first-line EGFR tyrosine kinase inhibitor or ALK inhibitor (lower score is better)
	89a: GCSF administered to patients who received chemotherapy for metastatic NSCLC cancer (lower score is better) (top 5 measure)

(continues)

TABLE C-6 National Standards in Support of AONN+ Metrics within Care Coordination/Care Transitions Domain *(continued)*

AONN+ METRIC: Percentage of navigated patients who adhere to institutional treatment pathways per quarter. (CO, ROI)	
Association	**Standard**
	90: PET or PET-CT ordered by the practice between 0 and 12 months after treatment with curative intent for patients with stage I or stage II NSCLC (lower score is better) (top 5 measure)
	91: Molecular testing for patients with stage IV NSCLC with adenocarcinoma histology
	NSCLC 92: Molecular testing turnaround time for patients with stage IV NSCLC with adenocarcinoma histology
	93: Concurrent chemoradiation for patients with a diagnosis of stage IIIB NSCLC
	90g: Operative report with documentation of residual disease within 48 hours of cytoreduction for women with invasive ovarian, fallopian tube, or peritoneal cancer
	91g: Complete staging for women with invasive stage I-IIIB ovarian, fallopian tube, or peritoneal cancer who have undergone cytoreduction
	92g: Intraperitoneal chemotherapy offered within 42 days of optimal cytoreduction to women with invasive stage III ovarian, fallopian tube, or peritoneal cancer
	93g: Intraperitoneal chemotherapy administered within 42 days of optimal cytoreduction to women with invasive stage III ovarian, fallopian tube, or peritoneal cancer
	94: Platin or taxane administered within 42 days following cytoreduction to women with invasive stage I (grade 3), IC-IV ovarian, fallopian tube, or peritoneal cancer. NQF endorsed #0218
	95: Venous thromboembolism (VTE) prophylaxis administered within 24 hours of cytoreduction to women with invasive ovarian, fallopian tube, or peritoneal cancer. NQF endorsed #0527
	96: Order for prophylactic parenteral antibiotic administration within 1-2 hours before cytoreduction for women with invasive ovarian, fallopian tube, or peritoneal cancer. NQF endorsed #0529
	97: Order for prophylactic parenteral antibiotic discontinuation within 24 hours after cytoreduction for women with invasive ovarian, fallopian tube, or peritoneal cancer
	111: PET, CT, or radionuclide bone scan ordered by practice within 2 months after diagnosis of early-stage prostate cancer with low risk of metastases (lower score is better) (top 5 test measure)
	112: PET, CT, or radionuclide bone scan ordered outside of practice within 2 months after diagnosis of early-stage prostate cancer with low risk of metastases (lower score is better) (top 5 test measure)

AONN+ METRIC: Percentage of navigated patients who adhere to institutional treatment pathways per quarter. (CO, ROI)	
Association	**Standard**
	113: Percentage of patients with a diagnosis of prostate cancer receiving androgen deprivation therapy (ADT) who received bone density testing to monitor for bone loss within 1 year of initiating ADT for prostate cancer (test measure)
	115: Percentage of patients with a diagnosis of prostate cancer receiving abiraterone for whom the medication is appropriately administered and monitored (test measure)
	Prostate 116: Percentage of patients with metastatic, hormone-sensitive prostate cancer who are offered docetaxel chemotherapy treatment within 4 months of initiation of hormone therapy (test measure). NQF 0387
	117: Percentage of patients, regardless of age, with a diagnosis of prostate cancer at high or very high risk of recurrence receiving external beam radiotherapy to the prostate who were prescribed adjuvant hormonal therapy (GnRH [gonadotropin-releasing hormone] agonist or antagonist). NQF 0390 small cell lung cancer (SCLC)
	118: Prophylactic cranial irradiation for patients with limited stage (LS) small cell lung cancer
	119: Overtreatment of SCLC patients with platinum-based chemotherapy
	SCLC 120: Early thoracic radiotherapy for patients with a diagnosis of limited stage SCLC
OCM	OCM-7: Prostate cancer: adjuvant hormonal therapy for high- or very high-risk prostate cancer
	OCM-8: Adjuvant chemotherapy is recommended or administered within 4 months (120 days) of diagnosis for patients under the age of 80 with AJCC III (lymph node-positive) colon cancer
	OCM-9: Combination chemotherapy is recommended or administered within 4 months (120 days) of diagnosis for women under 70 with AJCC T1c N0 M0, or stage 1B-III hormone receptor–negative breast cancer
	OCM-10: Trastuzumab administered to patients with AJCC stage 1 (T1c)-III and human epidermal growth factor receptor 2 (HER2)-positive breast cancer who receive adjuvant chemotherapy
	OCM-11: Breast cancer: hormonal therapy for stage 1 (T1b)-IIIC estrogen receptor/progesterone receptor (ER/PR)-positive breast cancer
	OCM-12: Documentation of current medications in the medical record

(continues)

TABLE C-6 National Standards in Support of AONN+ Metrics within Care Coordination/Care Transitions Domain   *(continued)*

AONN+ METRIC: Percentage of navigated patients who adhere to institutional treatment pathways per quarter. (CO, ROI)

Association	Standard
	OCM Primary Driver ■ Continuous improvement driven by data **OCM Secondary Driver** ■ Access and continuity: ability to obtain healthcare services in a timely manner ■ Care coordination: facilitation of care across the continuum, ensuring seamless transitions ■ Care planning and management: "coordinated plan that is evidence-based, integrated clinical care activities that are patient-specific and are agreed upon by the patient, caregivers, and clinician." Shared decision-making ■ Team-based care: comprehensive health services to individuals, families, and communities work in collaboration to meet patient needs and goals to achieve coordinated care across settings that equate high-quality care delivery ■ Data-driven quality improvement: "The use of a balanced set of measures with strong evidence base to inform change and practice transformation, identify and understand practice variation, provide clinical decision support, and monitor and sustain successful practices" ■ Evidence-based medicine: integration of clinical expertise, the patient's preferences or values, and the best research evidence to decide on the option that best suits the patient"
Quality Payment Program (QPP) The Merit-based Incentive Payment System (MIPS) Advanced Alternative Payment Models (Advanced APMs)	Colorectal cancer resection pathology reporting: pT category (primary tumor) and pN category (regional lymph nodes) with histologic grade. Measure ID: 100 Prostate cancer: avoidance of overuse of bone scan for staging low-risk prostate cancer patients. Measure ID: 102 Prostate cancer: adjuvant hormonal therapy for high-risk prostate cancer patients. Measure ID: 104 Preventive care and screening: screening for clinical depression and follow-up plan. Measure ID: 134 Melanoma: coordination of care. Measure ID: 138 Oncology: radiation dose limits to normal tissues. Measure ID: 156 Colonoscopy interval for patients with a history of adenomatous polyps—avoidance of inappropriate use—national quality strategy domain: communication and care coordination. Measure ID: 185 Oncology: cancer stage documented. Measure ID: 194

AONN + METRIC: Percentage of navigated patients who adhere to institutional treatment pathways per quarter. (CO, ROI)	
Association	**Standard**
	Melanoma: overutilization of imaging studies in melanoma. Measure ID: 224
	Quantitative immunohistochemical (IHC) evaluation of human epidermal growth factor receptor 2 testing (HER2) for breast cancer patients. Measure ID: 251
	Preoperative diagnosis of breast cancer. Measure ID: 263
	Sentinel lymph node biopsy for invasive breast cancer. Measure ID: 264
	Biopsy follow-up. Measure ID: 265
	Patient-centered surgical risk assessment and communication. Measure ID: 358
	Breast cancer: hormonal therapy for stage IC-IIIC estrogen receptor/progesterone receptor (ER/PR)-positive breast cancer. Measure ID: 71
	Prevention of central venous catheter-related bloodstream infections. Measure ID: 76
	Breast cancer resection pathology reporting: pT category (primary tumor) and pN category (regional lymph nodes) with histologic grade. Measure ID: 99
	Screening mammography cancer detection rate (CDR). Measure ID: ACRad 3
	Screening mammography invasive cancer detection rate (ICDR). Measure ID: ACRad 4
	Screening mammography abnormal interpretation rate (recall rate). Measure ID: ACRad 5
	Screening mammography positive predictive value 2 (PPV2 biopsy recommended). Measure ID: ACRad 6
	Composite procedural safety for central line placement. Measure ID: AQI 10
	Surgeon assessment for hereditary cause of breast cancer. Measure ID: American Society of Breast Surgeons (ASBS) 1
	Appropriate follow-up interval of 3 years recommended based on pathology findings from screening colonoscopy in average-risk patients. Measure ID: Gastro-Intestinal Quality Improvement Consortium (GIQIC) 15
	Prostate biopsy: proportion of patients undergoing a prostate biopsy with a PSA <4. Measure ID: Michigan Urological Surgical Improvement Collaborative (MUSIC) 8
	Ultrasound guidance for central line placement Measure. ID: THPSO 5
	Prostate cancer: avoidance of overuse of bone scan for staging low-risk prostate cancer patients. Measure ID: 102

(continues)

TABLE C-6 National Standards in Support of AONN+ Metrics within Care Coordination/Care Transitions Domain *(continued)*

AONN+ METRIC: Percentage of navigated patients who adhere to institutional treatment pathways per quarter. (CO, ROI)

Association	Standard
	Oncology: radiation dose limits to normal tissues. Measure ID: 156
	Radical prostatectomy pathology reporting. Measure ID: 250
	Lung cancer reporting (resection specimens). Measure ID: 396
	Hematology: myelodysplastic syndrome (MDS): documentation of iron stores in patients receiving erythropoietin therapy. Measure ID: 68
	Hematology: multiple myeloma: treatment with bisphosphonates. Measure ID: 69
	Breast cancer: hormonal therapy for stage IC-IIIC estrogen receptor/progesterone receptor (ER/PR)-positive breast cancer. Measure ID: 71
	Colon cancer: chemotherapy for AJCC stage III colon cancer patients. Measure ID: 72
	Prostate cancer: avoidance of overuse of CT scan for staging low-risk prostate cancer patients. Measure ID: MUSIC 3
	Prostate cancer: proportion of patients with low-risk prostate cancer receiving active surveillance. Measure ID: MUSIC 4
	Prostate cancer: percentage of prostate cancer cases with a length of stay >2 days. Measure ID: MUSIC 5
	Prostate biopsy: proportion of patients undergoing a repeat prostate biopsy within 12 months of their initial biopsy in the registry as a result of a finding of atypical small acinar proliferation (ASAP) as per the NCCN guidelines. Measure ID: MUSIC 9

AONN+ METRIC: Barriers to Care—number and list of specific barriers to care identified by navigator per month.* (PE, CO)

Association	Standard 2016
CoC	3.1: Patient Navigation Process
	A patient navigation process, driven by a triennial Community Needs Assessment, is established to address healthcare disparities and barriers to cancer care. Resources to address identified barriers may be provided either on-site or by referral
NAPBC	Standard 2.2: Patient Navigation
	A process is in place to guide the patient with breast abnormality through provided and referred services

AONN+ METRIC: Interventions—number of specific referrals/interventions offered to navigated patients per month.[†] (PE, CO)	
Association	**Standard**
QOPI	Pain assessed by second office visit. NQF endorsed #0383/#0384 (adapted)
	Pain intensity quantified by second office visit. NQF endorsed #0384 (adapted)
	Plan of care for moderate/severe pain documented. NQF endorsed #0383/#0384 (adapted)
	Pain addressed appropriately (defect-free measure 3, 4a, 5).* NQF endorsed #0383 (adapted)
	Pain assessed on either of the two most recent office visits. NQF endorsed #0383/#0384 (adapted)
	Pain intensity quantified on either of the two most recent office visits. NQF endorsed #0383/#0384 (adapted)
	6c: Plan of care for moderate/severe pain documented on either of the two most recent office visits. NQF endorsed #0383/#0384 (adapted)
	6d: Pain addressed appropriately on either of the two most recent office visits (defect-free measure, 6a, 6b, 6c). NQF endorsed #0383/#0384 (adapted)
	6e: Pain addressed appropriately by second office visit and during most recent office visits (defect-free measure 6 and 6d). NQF endorsed #0383/#0384 (adapted)
	8: Constipation assessed at time of narcotic prescription or following visit
	13oc5: Oral chemotherapy education provided prior to the start of therapy (defect-free measure 13oc5a-13oc5c)
	Core 13oc5a: Oral chemotherapy education provided prior to the start of therapy: missed doses
	13oc5b: Oral chemotherapy education provided prior to the start of therapy: toxicities
	13oc5c: Oral chemotherapy education provided prior to the start of therapy: clinic contact instructions
	21aa: Smoking status/tobacco use documented in past year.* NQF endorsed #0028 (adapted)
	22aa: Smoking/tobacco use cessation counseling recommended to smokers/tobacco users in past year. NQF endorsed #0028 (adapted)
	22bb: Tobacco cessation counseling administered or patient referred in past year. NQF endorsed #0028 (adapted)
	23aa: Smoking/tobacco use cessation administered appropriately in the past year (defect-free measure 21aa, 22aa, 22bb)
	33: Infertility risks discussed prior to chemotherapy with patients of reproductive age*

(continues)

AONN+ METRIC: Interventions—number of specific referrals/interventions offered to navigated patients per month.[†] (PE, CO)	
Association	**Standard**
	34: Fertility preservation options discussed or referral to specialist
	35: Pain assessed on either of the last two visits before death. NQF endorsed #0383/#0384 (adapted)
	EOL36a: Pain intensity quantified on either of the last two visits before death. NQF endorsed #0383/#0384 (adapted)
	EOL 37: Plan of care for moderate/severe pain documented on either of the last two visits before death. NQF endorsed #0383/#0384 (adapted)
	EOL 38: Pain addressed appropriately (defect-free measure 35, 36a, 37).* NQF endorsed #0383/#0384 (adapted)
	EOL 39: Dyspnea assessed on either of the last two visits before death
	EOL 40: Dyspnea addressed on either of the last two visits before death
	EOL 41: Dyspnea addressed appropriately (defect-free measure 39, 40)
OCM	OCM-4b: Oncology: Medical and Radiation—Plan of Care for Pain
	OCM Primary Driver
	■ Continuous improvement driven by data
	OCM Secondary Driver
	■ Access and continuity: ability to obtain healthcare serves in a timely manner
	■ Care coordination: facilitation of care across the continuum ensuring seamless transitions
	■ Care planning and management: "coordinated plan that is evidence-based, integrated clinical care activities that are patient-specific and are agreed upon by the patient, caregivers, and clinician." Shared decision-making
	■ Team-based care: comprehensive health services to individuals, families, and communities work in collaboration to meet patient needs and goals to achieve coordinated care across settings that equate high-quality care delivery
	■ Data-driven quality improvement: "The use of a balanced set of measures with strong evidence base to inform change and practice transformation, identify and understand practice variation, provide clinical decision support, and monitor and sustain successful practices"
	■ "Evidence-based medicine: "integration of clinical expertise, the patient's preferences or values, and the best research evidence to decide on the option that best suit the patient"
QPP MIPS Advanced APMs	Pain Assessment and Follow-Up. Measure ID: 131 Preventive care and screening: screening for clinical depression and follow-up plan. Measure ID: 134

AONN+ METRIC: Clinical Trial Education—number of patients educated on clinical trials by the navigator per month. (PE, CO)	
Association	**Standard 2016**
CoC	E9: Clinical research information eligibility requirement
	Standard 1.9: As appropriate to the cancer program category, the required percentages of patients are accrued to cancer-related clinical research studies each calendar year. The Clinical Research Coordinator documents and reports clinical research study enrollment information to the cancer committee annually
NAPBC	Standard 3.1: Clinical trial information about the availability of breast cancer–related clinical trials is provided to patients through a formal mechanism

AONN+ METRIC: Clinical Trial Referrals—number of navigated patients per month referred to clinical trial department. (PE, CO)	
Association	**Standard 2016**
CoC	Standard 1.9: As appropriate to the cancer program category, the required percentages of patients are accrued to cancer-related clinical research studies each calendar year. The Clinical Research Coordinator documents and reports clinical research study enrollment information to the cancer committee annually
NAPBC	Standard 3.2: Clinical trial accrual
	Two percent (2%) or more of all eligible breast cancer patients are accrued to treatment-related breast cancer clinical trials and/or research protocols annually

AONN+ METRIC: Patient Education—number of patient education encounters by navigator per month. (PE, CO, ROI)	
Association	**Standard**
NAPBC	Standard 2.17: culturally appropriate educational resources are available for patients along with the process to provide them. The materials are provided and reviewed on an annual basis and adjusted for the patient population

(continues)

AONN + METRIC: Patient Education—number of patient education encounters by navigator per month. (PE, CO, ROI)	
Association	**Standard**
	OCM-4b: Oncology: medical and radiation—plan of care for pain
	OCM Primary Driver
	▪ Continuous improvement driven by data
	OCM Secondary Driver
	▪ Access and continuity: ability to obtain healthcare serves in a timely manner
	▪ Care coordination: facilitation of care across the continuum, ensuring seamless transitions
	▪ Care planning and management: "coordinated plan that is evidence-based, integrated clinical care activities that are patient-specific and are agreed upon by the patient, caregivers, and clinician." Shared decision-making
	▪ Team-based care: comprehensive health services to individuals, families, and communities work in collaboration to meet patient needs and goals to achieve coordinated care across settings that equate high-quality care delivery
	▪ Data-driven quality improvement: "The use of a balanced set of measures with strong evidence base to inform change and practice transformation, identify and understand practice variation, provide clinical decision support, and monitor and sustain successful practices"
	▪ Evidence-based medicine: "integration of clinical expertise, the patient's preferences or values, and the best research evidence to decide on the option that best suits the patient"
QPP	Pain assessment and follow-up. Measure ID: 131
MIPS	Preventive care and screening: screening for clinical depression and follow-up plan. Measure ID: 134
Advanced	
APMs	Melanoma: coordination of care. Measure ID: 138

AONN + METRIC: Diagnosis to Initial Treatment—number of business days from diagnosis (date pathology resulted) to initial treatment modality (date of 1st treatment). (PE, CO)	
Association	**Standard**
CoC	Information can be monitored via CoC Cancer Quality Improvement Program (CQIP) report
	Days to First Treatment Quartiles Breast Cancer:
	0–17 days
	18–29 days
	30–44 days
	≥45 days

AONN + METRIC: Diagnosis to Initial Treatment—number of business days from diagnosis (date pathology resulted) to initial treatment modality (date of 1st treatment). (PE, CO)	
Association	**Standard**
QPP	Closing the referral loop: receipt of specialist report. Measure ID: 374
MIPS	Report turnaround time: radiography. Measure ID: ACRad 15
Advanced APMs	Report turnaround time: ultrasound (US) (excluding breast US). Measure ID: ACRad 16
	Report turnaround time: MRI. Measure ID; ACRad 17
	Report turnaround time: CT. Measure ID: ACRad 18
	Report turnaround time: PET. Measure ID: ACRad 19

* Obstacles that prevent a cancer patient from accessing care, services, resources, and/or support.
† The act of intervening, interfering, or interceding with the intent of modifying the outcome.

TABLE C-7 National Standards in Support of AONN + Metrics within Patient Empowerment, Patient Advocacy Domain

AONN + METRIC: Patient goals—percentage of analytic cases per month that patient goals identified and discussed with the navigator. (PE, CO, ROI)	
Association	**Standard**
QOPI	25a: Documentation of patient's advance directives by the third office visit
OCM	**OCM Primary Driver** Comprehensive, coordinated Cancer Care **OCM Secondary Drivers** ■ Care Planning and Management: "coordinated plan that is evidence-based, integrated clinical care activities that are patient-specific and are agreed upon by the patient, caregivers, and clinician." Shared decision -making ■ Patient and caregiver engagement: empowering patient and caregivers to engage in shared decision-making. Patient's health literacy is addressed
Quality Payment Program (QPP) The Merit-based Incentive Payment System (MIPS) Advanced Alternative Payment Models (Advanced APMs)	Advance care plan. Measure ID: 47 Discussion and shared decision-making surrounding treatment options. Measure ID: 390

TABLE C-8 National Standards in Support of AONN+ Metrics within Psychosocial Support, Assessment Domain

AONN+ METRIC: Psychosocial distress screening—number of navigated patients per month who received psychosocial distress screening at a pivotal medical visit with a validated tool.* (PE, CO)

Association	Standard
CoC	Standard 3.2: Psychosocial distress screening
	Each calendar year, the cancer committee develops and implements a process to integrate and monitor on-site psychosocial distress screening and referral for the provision of psychosocial care
	We utilize NCCN distress screening tool
	The following pivotal medical visits: CT simulation in radiation oncology, completion of radiation therapy, and chemo teach or first infusion in medical oncology. Identified "pivotal medical visits" are subject to revision as improvements to screening protocols are made
NAPBC	Standard 2.2: A patient navigation process is in place to guide the patient with a breast abnormality through provided and referred services
	Note: in the standard description it states in the definition of navigation that the navigator will provide individualized assistance offered to patients, families, and caregivers to help facilitate timely access to psychosocial care throughout the continuum of care.
	Standard 2.15: Support and rehabilitation services are provided or referred. Psychosocial distress screening and support
QOPI	24: Patient emotional well-being assessed by the second office visit
	25: Action taken to address problems with emotional well-being by the second office visit
	114: Percentage of patients with a diagnosis of prostate cancer (PC) with bone metastases who have a treatment plan to address pain documented at every physician/nurse practitioner/physician assistant visit (test measure)
	Certification Program Standard 1.4: Staff assesses and documents psychosocial concerns and need for support with each cycle or more frequently, with action taken when indicated.[†]
OCM	OCM-4a: Oncology: medical and radiation—pain intensity quantified
	OCM-5: Preventive care and screening: screening for depression and follow-up plan

AONN+ METRIC: Psychosocial distress screening—number of navigated patients per month who received psychosocial distress screening at a pivotal medical visit with a validated tool.* (PE, CO)	
Association	**Standard**
Quality Payment Program (QPP) The Merit-based Incentive Payment System (MIPS) Advanced Alternative Payment Models (Advanced APMs)	Pain assessment and follow-up. Measure ID: 131 Screening for clinical depression and follow-up plan. Measure ID: 134 Functional outcome assessment. Measure ID: 182 Depression utilization of the patient health questionnaire (PHQ-9) tool. Measure ID: 371 Depression screening. Measure ID: PPRNET 21 Quality of life (VR-12 or PROMIS Global-10) monitoring. Measure ID: OBERD 10

AONN+ METRIC: Social Support referrals—number of navigated patients referred to support network per month. (PE, CO, ROI)	
Association	**Standard 2016**
CoC	ACS serves on committee and reports on patient referrals to services, uninsured/Medicaid and service request per quarter
NAPBC	Standard 2.2: A patient navigation process is in place to guide the patient with a breast abnormality through provided and referred services Note: In the standard description it states in the definition of navigation that the navigator will provide individualized assistance offered to patients, families, and caregivers to help facilitate timely access to psychosocial care throughout the continuum of care. Connects patients and families to resources and support services. Standard 2.15: Support and rehabilitation services are provided or referred
QOPI	1.5: The healthcare setting provides information about financial resources and/or refers patients to psychosocial and other cancer support services
QPP MIPS Advanced APMs	Functional outcome assessment. Measure ID: 182 Tobacco use and help with quitting among adolescents. Measure ID: 402 Depression screening. Measure ID: PPRNET 21

* Pivotal medical visit definition: Period of high distress for the patient when psychosocial assessment should be completed. Define various validated tools as examples: Foundation for the Accreditation of Cellular Therapy (FACT), NCCN Psychosocial Distress Screening Thermometer.

† Psychosocial assessment: An evaluation of a person's mental health, social status, and functional capacity within the community. May include the use of a distress, depression, or anxiety screening form, patient self-report of distress, depression, or anxiety, or medical record documentation regarding patient coping, adjustment, depression, distress, anxiety, emotional status, family support and caregiving, coping style, cultural background, and socioeconomic status.

TABLE C-9 National Standards in Support of AONN+ Metrics within Survivorship and End-of-Life Domain

AONN+ METRIC: Survivorship care plan—number of navigated patients (patients with curative intent) per month who received a survivorship care plan and treatment summary. (PE, CO)

Association	Standard 2016
CoC	3.3: Survivorship Care Plan (SCP): A comprehensive SCP, including treatment summary. Follow American Society of Clinical Oncology (ASCO) template for patients with curative intent and who have completed therapy (other than hormonal). Cancer committee will develop a policy for the development and delivery of the SCP
NAPBC	2.20: Breast cancer survivorship care: a comprehensive breast cancer survivorship care process, SCP including a treatment summary given within 6 months of completing active treatment and no longer than 1 year from date of diagnosis. The survivorship care process is evaluated annually by the breast program leadership (BPL)
QOPI	17: Chemotherapy treatment summary completed within 3 months of chemotherapy treatment end
	18: Chemotherapy treatment summary provided to patient within 3 months of chemotherapy treatment end
	19: Chemotherapy treatment summary provided or communicated to practitioner(s) within 3 months of chemotherapy treatment end
	20: Chemotherapy treatment summary process completed within 3 months of chemotherapy end (defect-free measure 17, 18, 19)
	2.3: Patients are provided with verbal and written or electronic information as part of an education process before the first administration of treatment of each treatment plan. The content of this educational material will be documented
	2.3.3: Planned duration of treatment, schedule of treatment administration, drug names and supportive medications, drug-drug and drug-food interactions, and plan for missed doses
	2.3.4: Potential long-term and short-term adverse effects of therapy, including infertility risks for appropriate patients.
Quality Payment Program (QPP) The Merit-based Incentive Payment System (MIPS) Advanced Alternative Payment Models (Advanced APMs)	Patient self-management and action plan. Measure ID: AAAAI 14

AONN+ METRIC: Referrals to support services at the survivorship visit—number of navigated patients per month referred to appropriate support service at the survivorship visit. (PE, CO, ROI)	
Association	**Standard 2016**
CoC	ACS serves on committee and reports on patient referrals to services, uninsured/Medicaid and service request per quarter
NAPBC	Standard 2.2: A patient navigation process is in place to guide the patient with a breast abnormality through provided and referred services Note: In the standard description it states in the definition of navigation that the navigator will provide individualized assistance offered to patients, families, and caregivers to help facilitate timely access to psychosocial care throughout the continuum of care. Connects patients and families to resources and support services Standard 2.15: Support and rehabilitation services are provided or referred
QOPI	1.5: The healthcare setting provides information about financial resources and/or refers patients to psychosocial and other cancer support services.

AONN+ METRIC: Palliative care referral—number of navigated patients per month referred for palliative care service. (PE, CO, ROI)	
Association	**Standard**
CoC	Standard 2.4: Palliative care services Palliative care services are available to patients either on-site or by referral
NAPBC	Standard 2.15: Support and rehabilitation services are provided or referred—palliative care
QOPI	42: Hospice enrollment. NQF endorsed #0215 (adapted) EOL 43: Hospice enrollment or palliative care referral/services. NQF endorsed #0215 (adapted) 44: Hospice enrollment within 3 days of death (lower score is better). NQF endorsed #0216 (adapted) EOL 44a: Hospice enrollment and enrolled more than 3 days before death (defect-free measure 42, inverse 44). NQF endorsed #0216 (adapted)

(continues)

AONN + METRIC: Palliative care referral—number of navigated patients per month referred for palliative care service. (PE, CO, ROI)	
Association	**Standard**
	45: Hospice enrollment within 7 days of death (lower score is better). NQF endorsed #0216 (adapted) EOL
	45a: Hospice enrollment and enrolled more than 7 days before death (defect-free measure 42, inverse 45).* NQF endorsed #0216 (adapted)
	46: For patients not referred, hospice or palliative care discussed within the last 2 months of life. NQF endorsed #0215 (adapted) EOL
	47: Hospice enrollment, palliative care referral/services, or documented discussion (combined measure, 43 or 46). NQF endorsed
	98: Pain quantified using a standardized instrument at every clinical encounter in the past 3 months for patients with advanced/metastatic lung, pancreatic, and colorectal cancer
	99: Plan of care for pain when moderate/severe pain present in the past 3 months for patients with advanced/metastatic lung, pancreatic, and colorectal cancer
	100: Constipation, fatigue, and nausea assessed at the clinic visit following a new prescription or increasing opioid regimen for patients with advanced/metastatic lung, pancreatic, and colorectal cancer
	101: Dyspnea assessed on every clinic visit in the past 3 months for patients with advanced/metastatic lung, pancreatic, and colorectal cancer
	102: Dyspnea addressed, if present, in the past 3 months for patients with advanced/metastatic lung, pancreatic, and colorectal cancer (test measure)
	103: Nausea and vomiting assessed on every clinic visit in the past 3 months for patients with advanced/metastatic lung, pancreatic, and colorectal cancer
	104: Nausea and vomiting addressed, when present, in the past 3 months for patients with advanced/metastatic lung, pancreatic, and colorectal cancer (test measure)
	105: Performance status assessed at every clinic visit in the past 3 months for patients with advanced/metastatic lung, pancreatic, and colorectal cancer
	106: Emotional well-being assessed within first 2 visits after diagnosis with advanced/metastatic lung, pancreatic, and colorectal cancer
	107: Emotional well-being assessed within 2 visits of changes in clinical status for patients with advanced lung, pancreatic, and colorectal cancer
	108: Documented substance abuse history, including tobacco, alcohol, and illicit drug use, within the first 3 visits after diagnosis with advanced/metastatic lung, pancreatic, and colorectal cancer (test measure)

AONN+ METRIC: Palliative care referral—number of navigated patients per month referred for palliative care service. (PE, CO, ROI)	
Association	**Standard**
	109: Advance directive documentation within first 3 visits after diagnosis with advanced/metastatic lung, pancreatic, and colorectal cancer (test measure)
	110: Hospice recommended and no chemotherapy with performance status 3 or 4 for patients with advanced/metastatic lung, pancreatic, and colorectal cancer (test measure)
OCM	OCM-3: Proportion of patients who died who were admitted to hospice for 3 days or more (loosely fits with this measure)
QPP MIPS Advanced APMs	Quality of life (VR-12 or PROMIS Global-10) monitoring. Measure ID: OBERD 10

TABLE C-10 National Standards in Support of AONN+ Metrics within Professional Roles and Responsibilities Domain

AONN+ METRIC: Oncology navigator annual core competencies review—percentage of staff members who have completed institutionally developed navigator core competencies annually to validate core knowledge of oncology navigation. (CO)	
Association	**Standard**
CoC	Standard 1.10: Clinical educational activity
	The activity is focused on the use of AJCC or other appropriate staging in clinical practice, which includes the use of appropriate prognostic indicators and evidence-based national guidelines used in treatment planning
NAPBC	Standard 2.14: Nursing care is provided by nurses with specialized knowledge and skills in diseases of the breast
	Standard 5.1: Members of the Breast Care Team participate in a minimum of two local, state, regional, or national breast-specific continuing medical education (or equivalent) activities annually
	If patient navigation is provided by a lay navigator, then he or she is required to have documented patient navigation training

TABLE C-11 National Standards in Support of AONN+ Metrics within Operations Management, Organizational Development, Health Economics Domain

AONN+ METRIC: 30-, 60-, 90-day readmission rate*	
Association	**Standard 2016**
QOPI	49ed: Percentage of patients who died from cancer with more than one emergency department visit in the last 30 days of life (lower score is better). NQF endorsed #0211
	49icu: Percentage of patients who died from cancer admitted to the Intensive Care Unit (ICU) in the last 30 days of life (lower score is better). NQF endorsed #0213
OCM	OCM-1: Risk-adjusted proportion of patients with all-cause hospital admissions within 6-month episode
	Primary Driver
	Management of OCM payments
	Secondary Driver
	Strategic use of revenue—implementation of performance improvement to use the payments to enhance services and maintain infrastructure and resources
Quality Payment Program (QPP)	Unplanned hospital admission. Measure ID: 19
The Merit-based Incentive Payment System (MIPS)	Lung cancer reporting (biopsy/cytology specimens). Measure ID: 395
	Melanoma reporting. Measure ID: 397
Advanced Alternative Payment Models (Advanced APMs)	Unplanned 30-day re-operation after mastectomy. Measure ID: ASBS 7
	Unplanned hospital readmission within 30 days of principal procedure. Measure ID: AQI 26
	Mean length of stay for inpatients—all patients. Measure ID: HCPR 2
	30-day all-cause re-admission rate for all discharged inpatients. Measure. ID: HCPR 6
	Extended length of stay (LOS). Measure ID: MBS 7
	Unplanned hospital re-admission within 30 days of principal procedure. Measure ID: MBS 9
	30-day re-admission for pneumonia. Measure ID: PInc 3
	Unplanned hospital admission. Measure ID: QUANTUM 19
	Unplanned ICU admission measure ID: QUANTUM 20

AONN+ METRIC: Referrals to revenue-generating services[†]	
Association	**Standard**
CoC	ACS serves on committee and reports on patient referrals to services, uninsured/Medicaid and service request per quarter
	Standard 3.1: Patient navigation process
	A patient navigation process, driven by a triennial community needs assessment, is established to address healthcare disparities and barriers to cancer care. Resources to address identified barriers may be provided either on-site or by referral
	Standard 2.3: Genetic counseling and risk assessment
	Cancer risk assessment, genetic counseling, and genetic testing services are provided to patients either on-site or by referral to a qualified genetics professional
	Standard 2.4: Palliative care services
	Palliative care services are available to patients either on-site or by referral
NAPBC	Standard 2.2: A patient navigation process is in place to guide the patient with a breast abnormality through provided and referred services
	Standard 2.15: Support and rehabilitation services are provided or referred. Psychosocial distress screening and support
	Standard 2.16: Genetic evaluation and management: cancer risk assessment, genetic counseling, and genetic testing services are provided or referred
QOPI	65: Genetic testing addressed appropriately for patients with invasive colorectal cancer (defect-free measure 65a–65c)
	65a: Genetic counseling, referral for counseling, or genetic testing for patients with invasive colorectal cancer with increased hereditary risk of colorectal cancer
	65b: Patient consent for genetic testing ordered by the practice for patients with invasive colorectal cancer
	65c: Patient with invasive colorectal cancer counseled, or referred for counseling, to discuss results following genetic testing
QPP MIPS Advanced APMs	Surgeon assessment for hereditary cause of breast cancer. Measure ID: ASBS 1

AONN+ METRIC: Emergency department utilization[‡]	
Association	**Standard**
OCM	OCM-2: Risk-adjusted proportion of patients with all-cause ED visits who did not result in a hospital admission within the 6-month episode
	Primary Driver
	Management of OCM payments
	Secondary Driver
	Strategic use of revenue—implementation of performance improvement to use the payments to enhance services and maintain infrastructure and resources
QPP	Three-day return rate ED. Measure ID: American College of Emergency Physicians (ACEP) 12
MIPS	
Advanced APMs	Three-day all-cause return ED visit rate—all patients. Measure ID: Adjusted Community Rate Proposal (ECPR) 11
	Three-day all-cause return ED visit rate—adults. ECPR 12
	Three-day all-cause return ED visit rate—pediatrics. Measure ID: ECPR 13
	Three-day all-cause return ED visit rate with placement into inpatient or observation status on re-visit. Measure ID: ECPR 17
	Mean time from emergency department (ED) arrival to ED departure for pediatric ED patients placed into inpatient or observation status. Measure ID: ECPR 10
	Door to diagnostic evaluation by a provider—adult emergency department (ED) patients. Measure ID: ECPR 2
	Door to diagnostic evaluation by a provider—pediatric emergency department (ED) patients. Measure ID: ECPR 3
	Mean time from emergency department (ED) arrival to ED departure for all discharged ED patients. Measure ID: ECPR 4
	Mean time from emergency department (ED) arrival to ED departure for discharged lower acuity ED patients. Measure ID: ECPR 5
	Mean time from emergency department (ED) arrival to ED departure for discharged higher acuity ED patients. Measure ID: ECPR 6
	Mean time from emergency department (ED) arrival to ED departure for all ED patients placed into inpatient or observation status. Measure ID: ECPR 8
	Mean time from emergency department (ED) arrival to ED departure for adult ED patients placed into inpatient or observation status. Measure ID: ECPR 9
	Mean time from emergency department (ED) arrival to ED departure for all ED patients placed into inpatient or observation status. Measure ID: HCPR 1
	Unplanned emergency room (ER) visits. Measure ID: MBS 8
	Median time from ED arrival to ED departure for admitted ED patients. Measure ID: PInc 29
	Admit decision time to ED departure time for admitted patients. Measure ID: PInc 30
	Median time from ED arrival to ED departure for discharged ED Patients. Measure ID: PInc 31

AONN+ METRIC: No-show rate—number of navigated patients who do not complete a scheduled appointment per month. (ROI)	
Association	**Standard**
QOPI	2.3.11: The missed appointment policy of the healthcare setting and expectations for rescheduling or cancelling

AONN+ METRIC: Emergency admissions per number of chemotherapy patients[§]	
Association	**Standard 2016**
OCM	OCM-2: Risk-adjusted proportion of patients with all-cause ED visits that did not result in a hospital admission within the 6-month episode
	Primary Driver Management of OCM payments
	Secondary Driver Strategic use of revenue—implementation of performance improvement to use the payments to enhance services and maintain infrastructure and resources

*Number of navigated patients readmitted to the hospital at 30, 60, and 90 days. Report quarterly. Measures return on investment.
[†]Number of referrals to revenue-generating services per month by navigator. Measures return on investment.
[‡]Number of navigated patients visits to the emergency room per month. Measures return on investment.
[§]Number of navigated patient visits per 1,000 chemotherapy patients who had an emergency room visit per month. Measures return on investment.

TABLE C-12 National Standards in Support of AONN+ Metrics within Research, Quality, Performance Improvement Domain

AONN+ METRIC: Patient experience/patient satisfaction with care—patient experience or patient satisfaction survey results per month.* (PE)	
Association	**Standard**
OCM	OCM-6: Patient-reported experience
Quality Payment Program (QPP) The Merit-based Incentive Payment System (MIPS) Advanced Alternative Payment Models (Advanced APMs)	Composite patient experience measure. Measure ID: AQI 11 Quality of life (VR-12 or PROMIS Global-10) monitoring. Measure ID: OBERD 10 Current Group Consumer Assessment of Healthcare Providers & Systems (CG-CAHPS) adult visit composite tracking. Measure ID: OBERD 12 CG-CAHPS patient rating. Measure ID: OBERD 17

AONN+ METRIC: Navigation program validation based on community needs assessment—monitor one major goal of current navigation program annually as defined by cancer committee Example: Population served. (PE, CO, ROI)	
Association	**Standard 2016**
CoC	Standard 3.1: Patient navigation process A patient navigation process, driven by a triennial community needs assessment, is established to address healthcare disparities and barriers to cancer care. Resources to address identified barriers may be provided either on-site or by referral

* Utilize institution-specific navigation tool with internal benchmark.

The metrics in **TABLE C-13** do not specifically align with the national standards and indicators. However, AONN+ believes these to be important metrics to collect for a navigation program to demonstrate value and sustainability.

TABLE C-13 AONN+ Standardized Metrics Not Captured in National Standards and Indicators Crosswalk

Domain	Metric
Operations Management, Organizational Development, Health Economics	**Navigation Operational Budget—Monthly operating expenses by line item. (ROI)** Definition: Operational budget is a combination of known expenses, expected future costs, and forecasted income over the course of a year **Navigation Caseload—Number of new cases, open cases, and closed cases navigated per month. (ROI)** New cases: New patient cases referred to the navigation program per month Open cases: Patient cases that remain open/month Closed cases: Number of patient cases closed per month. Formal closing of patient cases from the navigation program **Patient Retention Through Navigation—Number of analytic cases per month or quarter that remained in your institution due to navigation. (ROI)**
Care Coordination/Care Transition	**Diagnosis to 1st Oncology Consult—Number of business days from diagnosis (date pathology resulted) to initial oncology consult (date of 1st appointment). (PE, CO)**

Domain	Metric
Community Outreach and Education	**Completion of Diagnostic Workup—Number of navigated individuals with abnormal screening that completed diagnostic workup per month/quarter. (CO, ROI)** **Disparate Population at Screening Event—Number of individuals per quarter at community screening events by Office of Management and Budget Standards. (PE, CO)** Disparate population definition: The National Institute on Minority Health and Health Disparities defines disparities as differences in the incidence, prevalence, mortality, and burden of disease and other adverse health conditions that exist among specific populations in the United States (racial and ethnic minorities, low socioeconomic status)
Patient Empowerment/Patient Advocacy	**Caregiver Support—Number of caregiver needs/ preferences discussed with navigator per month. (CO)** **Identify Learning Style Preference—Number of navigated patients per month whose preferred learning style was discussed during the intake process. (PE, CO)** Learning styles: ■ Visual (spatial): You prefer using pictures, images, and spatial understanding ■ Aural (auditory-musical): You prefer using sound and music ■ Verbal (linguistic): You prefer using words, both in speech and writing ■ Physical (kinesthetic): You prefer using your body, hands, and sense of touch ■ Logical (mathematical): You prefer using logic, reasoning, and systems ■ Social (interpersonal): You prefer to learn in groups or with other people ■ Solitary (intrapersonal): You prefer to work alone and use self-study
Professional Roles and Responsibilities	**Navigation Knowledge at time of Orientation— Percentage of new hires who have completed institutionally developed navigator core competencies. (CO)**

(continues)

TABLE C-13 AONN + Standardized Metrics Not Captured in National Standards and Indicators Crosswalk *(continued)*

Domain	Metric
Research and Performance Improvement	**Patient Transitions from Point of Entry—Percentage of navigated analytic cases per month transitioned from institutional point of entry to initial treatment modality. (PE, CO)** Care Transitions Definition: "The movement patients make between healthcare practitioners and settings as their condition and care needs change during the course of chronic or acute illness"* Define modality: chemotherapy, surgery, radiation therapy, endocrine therapy, and biotherapy **Diagnostic Workup to Diagnosis—Number of business days from date of abnormal finding to pathology report for navigated patients. (CO))**
Survivorship/End of Life	**Transition from Treatment to Survivorship— Percentage of navigated analytic cases per month transitioned from completed cancer treatment to survivorship. (PE, CO)** Care Transitions Definition: "The movement patients make between healthcare practitioners and settings as their condition and care needs change during the course of chronic or acute illness"*

* Coleman EA. The Care Transitions Program. Aurora, CO: Division of Health Care Policy and Research, University of Colorado Denver; February 8, 2013. www.caretransitions.org.

For additional information, please visit www.jons-online.com/issue-archive/2017-issues/may-2017-vol-8-no-5.

Keep in mind that the references to the CoC will require adjusting since the standards of care numbers are changing with the revision of the standards due to go into effect in 2020.

Appendix D

Resources

AONN+'s official website: www.aonnonline.org

Shockney, L. *Team-Based Oncology Care: The Pivotal Role of Oncology Navigation.* 1st ed. New York, NY: Springer, 2018.

Toolkit from Pfizer on navigation in cancer care: http://s3.amazonaws.com/pfizerpro.com/assets/patientnavigation.com/Patient_Navigation_in_Cancer_Care_2.0_%C2%ADWebsite_12.04.18.pdf

Appendix E

Glossary

https://aonnonline.org/education/helpful-definitions

▶ Community Outreach

Community outreach is the practice of conducting local public awareness activities through targeted community interaction. In cancer, community outreach frequently seeks to encourage early screening and detection for different malignancies, include breast cancer, colorectal cancer, melanoma, and other tumor types

▶ Continuity of Care

The provision of healthcare services to patients in a coordinated manner and without disruption despite involvement of different practitioners in different care settings.

▶ Distress

Emotional, social, spiritual, or physical pain or suffering that may cause a wide range of feelings as patients cope with their cancer diagnosis and treatment. Patients experience distress along a continuum, which ranges from normal adjustment through diagnosable mental disorders. Nurse Navigators should monitor patient distress levels to make sure that adequate psychosocial resources are made available.

▶ Navigation Process

Helping patients overcome health care system barriers and providing them with timely access to quality medical and psychosocial care from before cancer diagnosis through all phases of their cancer experience.

▶ Nurse Navigator

A clinically trained individual responsible to identify and address barriers to timely and appropriate cancer treatment. They guide the patient through the cancer care continuum from diagnosis through survivorship. More specifically, the nurse navigator acts as a central point of contact for a patient and coordinates all components involved in cancer care including surgical, medical, and radiation oncologists; social workers; patient education; community support; financial and insurance assistance; etc. This person has the clinical background and is a critical member of the multidisciplinary cancer team.

▶ Palliative Care

Specialized medical care to prevent or treat the symptoms and side effects of the disease and treatment with a goal of improving overall quality of life. Palliative care should be offered to cancer patients at the time of diagnosis through survivorship or end of care. The goal of palliative care is not to cure, but to provide supportive care and symptom management as early as possible.

▶ Patient or Non-Clinically Licensed Navigator

An individual who does not have or use clinical training to provide individualized assistance to patients and families affected by cancer to improve access to health care services. A patient navigator may work within the health care system at point of screening, diagnosis, treatment or survivorship or across the cancer care spectrum or outside the health care system at a community based organization or as a freelance patient navigator. The patient navigator, unlike a "lay" navigator is a paid professional and serves as a broker between the patient and the health care system.

The patient navigator is a primary point of contact for the patient and works with other members of the care team to coordinate care for the patient. This critical person on the multidisciplinary team provides important perspective on logistical, structural and social needs of the patient as well as cultural considerations, patient values and care preferences. In general, a patient navigator provides assistance with identifying challenges to cancer care, identifying potential solutions with patients and families, identifying financial assistance to address patient needs, helping patients identify priority questions about their care, helping patients use time effectively with clinical providers and working with social work and nurse navigator colleagues to provide psychosocial and community support. A social worker or nurse may perform the role of a patient navigator, but in this instance they should discuss their scope of practice with their supervisor to ensure they perform duties within their hired role as opposed to within their clinical training.

▶ Psychosocial Distress Screening

The use of a brief tool to identify patients at greatest risk for an unpleasant experience of a psychological (cognitive, behavioral, emotional), social, and/or spiritual nature that may interfere with the ability to cope effectively with cancer, its physical symptoms, and its treatment. Referral for further assessment and/or to community resources for information and support along with follow-up to see if distress is reduced is key.

▶ Quality of Life

An assessment of the patient's ability to have an enjoyable and fulfilling life. Quality of life (QOL) is a measurement of the patient's well-being, including mental status, stress level, sexual function, self-perceived health status, and ability to perform activities of daily living. Nurse Navigators must be aware of factors, such as medical treatments, that may impair or improve a patient's quality of life

▶ Survivorship

Cancer survivorship refers to anyone who has been diagnosed with cancer. Survivorship starts at the time of disease diagnosis and continues throughout the rest of the patient's life.

▶ Survivorship Care Plan

An individualized care plan for patients for patients who have been treated for cancer. The survivorship care plan includes guidelines for monitoring and maintaining patient health.

Index

Note: Page numbers followed by "*f*" and "*t*" indicate figures and tables, respectively.

U

utilization management (UM), 18–19
utilization review (UR), 18

V

volunteer navigator, 48

W

webinars, 89
website, 90–92
What Would Lillie Do? (WWLD?), 89